THE DYING PATIENT

GW00703458

The Dying Patient

EDITED BY

RONALD W RAVEN

OBE, OStJ, TD, MD(Hon), FRCS

Member of Council, Royal College of Surgeons of England;
late Hunterian Professor, Arris and Gale Lecturer and Erasmus Wilson Demonstrator;
Bradshaw Lecturer, Royal College of Surgeons of England;
Consulting Surgeon, Westminster Hospital;
Consulting Surgeon, Royal Marsden Hospital and Institute of Cancer Research;
Consulting Surgeon, Star and Garter Home for Disabled Sailors, Soldiers and Airmen;
Chairman, Marie Curie Memorial Foundation

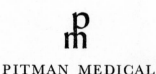

PITMAN MEDICAL

First published 1975

Pitman Medical Publishing Co Ltd
42 Camden Road, Tunbridge Wells,
Kent TN1 2QD

Associated Companies

UNITED KINGDOM
Pitman Publishing Ltd, London
Focal Press Ltd, London

USA
Pitman Publishing Corporation, New York
Fearon Publishers Inc, California

AUSTRALIA
Pitman Publishing Pty Ltd, Melbourne

CANADA
Pitman Publishing, Toronto
Copp Clark Publishing, Toronto

EAST AFRICA
Sir Isaac Pitman and Sons Ltd, Nairobi

SOUTH AFRICA
Pitman Publishing Co SA (Pty) Ltd, Johannesburg

ISBN 272 79354 X
Cat. No. 21 3201 81

Printed in Great Britain by
Clarke, Doble & Brendon Ltd, Plymouth

Contents

List of Contributors

Preface

CARING FOR dying patients and giving sympathetic support to bereaved families are profoundly important parts of the work of doctors, nurses, ministers and other members of the caring professions. Suitable adequate instruction is therefore required during their training, fitting them to deal with these difficult and delicate problems throughout their professional lives. There is general agreement that this subject has not received adequate study, but it is now attracting increasing attention, which is deserved. Much is learned about this special kind of care in hospital, hospice, nursing home and family home by unhurried observation of, and discussion with, patients and relatives, where a thoughtful, sympathetic approach is essential. To give as well as to receive, sensitivity of mind and warmth of heart are basic requirements, which are enhanced by personal experience of sorrow and suffering. An immense contribution can be made to the quality of family life under this stress and strain by those who have prepared themselves to give it.

Reading this book will undoubtedly prove helpful for many people, including those working in the caring professions and others wishing to know more about this subject. The chapter headings reveal the wide coverage and each chapter forms a distinct entity. The book was actually designed with this objective in view, so that if a reader wished to know about children or elderly people, or the relief of pain, for example, the appropriate chapter is available for study. In the complete text there is a definite overlap of information, but this is not caused by editorial failure. In fact the opposite is true, for the Editor purposely elected not to delete any repetitive material as he preferred to keep each chapter as a complete whole. This applies particularly to the attitudes of the authors to the different sub-sections, which is understandable, for they have similar beliefs and skills. In the general care of these patients and families by different professionals there is much in common, and even the use of some of the same medicines is discussed in different chapters.

There can be no doubt that many students, especially medical, nursing, social welfare and ordinands, require instruction, both theoretical and practical, to care for patients who are dying. When all is said and done, however, it is the individual professional that matters most; what he or she believes and stands for in life. Individual faith and adherence to fundamental beliefs are of paramount importance when visiting the fatally sick and bereaved, who have much they wish to discuss and perhaps doubts to solve and fears to allay.

I count it a privilege to be the Editor of this book and feel very grateful to the authors who have contributed such helpful chapters, and the publisher, especially Mr. Stephen Neal, for his collaboration. I feel sure I speak for all who have taken part in its publication when I say that we shall be satisfied if the book brings help and comfort to those who need this support in a very delicate and perhaps difficult situation.

RONALD W. RAVEN

I

Relief in Death and Bereavement

RONALD W. RAVEN

THE WHOLE animated creation, which includes mankind, is subject to the experience of physical death. The records of the beginnings of human history attest that, even at that early stage of his life upon earth, man was reminded of the inevitability of his death (Gen. 2: 17). Later there emerged in the *Old Testament* writings, the belief that death is a state or condition with an existence for man beyond the grave, however difficult this may be to describe or quantify. The conviction exists in man that death is not the end of everything, but a whisper of immortality can be heard as expressed by Tennyson, 'tis life not death for which we pant'.

Flashes of this conscious hope occur in many ancient writings. For example, Job had no doubt about immortality, and succinctly expressed his belief for our encouragement (Job 19: 26). In the *New Testament* Jesus illuminated this dark subject by not speaking of death as a physical experience but stressed the certainty of a fuller life hereafter. Neither did He offer us any explanation of this great mystery, but only called attention to the fact of death in using these expressions—'taste of death' (Mark 9: 1) and 'see death' (John 8: 51). He also held out to us the welcome prospect that whosoever believes in Him shall 'never die' (John 11: 26). Jesus endured physical death Himself and emerged triumphant in resurrection, and on numerous occasions during His ministry He called our attention to the certainty that all who believe in Him will enjoy Resurrection Life with Him on the other side of death.

The Lord Jesus relieves further our apprehension of physical death by His description of death as a sleep (Mark 5: 39; John 11: 11). This conception has brought comfort and consolation to people in all generations from the early Christian era to the present day. On the occasion of the miracle of raising Lazarus from the dead, Our Lord clearly showed His conception of physical death (John 11: 1–45). He understands human feelings about death and the dismay caused by the severance of spirit from body. Few can really face this prospect with equanimity, especially when time is given to contemplate it happening. Neither can we remain immune from deep sorrow when in the presence of death affecting family, friend or patient. We then become conscious of the real mysteries of life and fellowship with God, who is Life. Our Lord demonstrated that death is not final and the certainty of physical resurrection in this miracle. He did not use even the dreaded word 'death', but spoke of sleep and wakening out of sleep; whilst giving faith and hope to those who were bereaved and comfort in their sorrow. In the raising of Lazarus from the dead we learn the truth that He is the Resurrection and the Life and can see the reality of His own resurrection after the Crucifixion. By dying, Jesus broke the power of death and we can truly say, 'though I walk through the valley of the shadow of death, I will fear no evil, for Thou art with me' (Ps. 23: 4). This doctrine of the resurrection stands at the centre of the Christian faith.

Our Lord's view of death was developed further by St Paul, who wrote of 'them also which sleep in Jesus'. (1 Thess. 4: 13–14). The realisation that a completed life is rounded off by such a sleep gives peace to troubled minds, which is enhanced with the realisation of the awakening to follow. The *New Testament* writers continually reaffirmed their confidence in the resurrection of the body. Faith in this physical resurrection gives us hope in the future, and those who sorrow are exhorted by St Paul to 'comfort one another with these words' (1 Thess. 4: 18).

It is not my purpose here to discuss the Johannine and Pauline writings concerning spiritual death, which they described as the condition of man resulting from sin, for I am writing here about physical death.

In my professional work I have proved how much comfort and hope are engendered by these immutable truths. In the human extremity of physical death only faith in the love and power of God is competent to sustain us. Then we become conscious of spiritual power which can be communicated to others in need of this help. The doctor has the responsibility of caring for the physical needs of the dying patient and is given the privilege of giving comfort by a meaningful touch, encouraging words, or a prayer. Patients can understand their mystic meaning although little may be spoken. Time and concentration are required for this special service for others. The doctor must also have faith in the risen Christ and have overcome thereby the personal fear of death.

The care of patients during their final illnesses over various periods of time is a privilege, for they greatly appreciate the visits of the doctor and realise they are not forgotten. They may be cared for in hospitals, nursing homes, or family homes and require numerous medical and nursing skills according to the particular illness. Symptoms are treated so that the patient remains free from pain and in comfort. Much nursing care is required by some patients, especially those who are paralysed in various ways. The details of the treatments are given in other chapters of this book and so are not repeated here. Death may occur quite suddenly, causing shock to the family, but many patients suffer the effects of a chronic illness requiring fortitude by all the members of the family.

I have the responsibility of caring for many patients with various cancerous diseases; this particular diagnosis understandably causes unrest and anxiety to the patient and family. Various questions require answering at all stages of these illnesses. An explanation about the treatment and prognosis is given to the family, with the assurance that everything will be done to help the patient throughout the illness. When adequate time is given for these discussions confident professional relationships are established, which help everybody. The question whether the patient should be told he or she has a cancerous disease needs some discussion. Information is given with sympathetic understanding of the situation and in the kindest way, in the presence of a near relative. Words are chosen carefully to engender faith and confidence, and nothing should be said to take away a patient's hope. I believe we can work professionally in a more helpful way when patients are told about the illness, and by understanding something about the problems to be solved they can co-operate more usefully.

I never feel able to answer the questions about the length of time the patient is likely to live, except when the end is obviously near, and I explain that all our lives are in the hand of God. Thus, when a patient enquires about his illness, I feel it is right to discuss the situation along these lines. Sometimes the family specifically requests that no mention is made of the diagnosis to the patient to avoid any upset. I respect their wishes, although work may be made more difficult when a patient realises the gradual deterioration of health without a real explanation being given. During the final days of the illness I indicate to the family that time is becoming short for the patient, and I believe that the majority of these patients know about their condition so that only a little explanation is necessary. It is important to keep the patient's trust and say nothing to undermine his confidence in the doctor.

The whole family require help at these times to ameliorate the strains and stresses caused by chronic illnesses. Even relationships between parents, and parents and children, can become unhappy. An unhappy situation is created when seriously ill children with a short life expectancy are brought by their parents over long distances for treatment. When they come with hope it is a hard task to explain that active treatment might even be injurious in a terminal state. I am always impressed by the courage and calmness of these children in their weakness.

Patients who are seriously ill and cannot recover and their families, appreciate the frequent visits of the doctor, who can give much sympathetic help and support to ameliorate the sorrow and suffering which become more intense as death approaches for the loved relation. The presence of the doctor who has become a trusted friend during the illness is a source of solace to them in their grief. A special, unhurried visit following soon after the patient's death to talk and discuss is greatly appreciated by the family. These visits to the bereaved family should continue for a further period of time, until there is an amelioration of their grief and loneliness, which can be almost too great to bear.

In these distressful circumstances expressions of Christian faith give courage and hope and bring healing of the spirit. We can be sure that God is always ready to help us in our need, for when Jesus prayed in Gethsemane for relief from His anguish of approaching death, an angel was sent from heaven to strengthen Him in His hour of extreme physical and spiritual suffering. Although this suffering was not removed, He was given grace and strength to bear it, just as many of us have experienced that divine strength.

Members of the healing professions will continue to work for the good of the afflicted throughout the world, and in this way each generation makes its own contribution to human welfare and relief, until the day breaks and the shadows of suffering fly away, when God will decisively and finally intervene in the lives of men.

This eternal deliverance from sorrow and suffering is described in the words of St John the Divine: 'And God shall wipe away all tears from their eyes; and there shall be no more death, neither sorrow, nor crying, neither shall there be any more pain . . .' (Rev. 21: 4).

2

The Seriously Ill Child

LINDY BURTON

UNTIL QUITE RECENTLY it was not uncommon for a family to be faced with the task of caring for a seriously ill child. Often such children suffered from infectious diseases, whose onset was sudden and whose course was swift. Adequate treatment procedures were lacking and the lives of affected children were correspondingly brief. Care was essentially palliative and concentrated solely on the young patient's physical needs. Today, by contrast, advances in medical knowledge and improvements in nutrition and domestic hygiene, have reduced significantly the more common childhood complaints,[1] and improved the quality and length of life of most children.[2]

Whilst such progress is an obvious source of satisfaction, it is not without disadvantages. In the midst of generally well peers, the child with a serious illness may now feel lonely and different, unable to participate in an increasingly competitive world. What is more, he may be forced to endure this limbo state for many years, maintained in variable health by improved treatment

[1]For example, there has been a significant decline in child mortality due to infections. In 1931, over 2,000 children per million, aged 1–14 years, died of infectious diseases in the United Kingdom, as compared with under 100 for a similar population in 1970 (Meadow and Smithells, 1973).
[2]Mortality in childhood is highest during the first year of life. Taking the infant mortality rate (number of deaths per 1,000 live births) for the United Kingdom it is seen that the infant death rate has now fallen to one tenth of the level observed at the turn of the century.
Between 1906–1910 117·1 infants died in the first year of life
        1926–1930 67·6 infants died in the first year of life
        1946–1950 36·3 infants died in the first year of life
        1956–1960 22·6 infants died in the first year of life
        1966–1970 18·4 infants died in the first year of life
(Figures taken from the Statistical Review of the Registrar General for England and Wales, 1970).

techniques.[1] Unless those who care for the sick child appreciate, and attempt to assuage, the numerous emotional, social, and intellectual problems which protracted illness cause, his days may be blighted by the shadow of death, rather than lived joyfully and to the full.

FACTORS AFFECTING THE CHILD'S RESPONSE TO HIS SERIOUS ILLNESS

Many factors affect the way in which a child responds to serious illness. Some of the most crucial are his age and level of development, the nature of his symptoms, the degree of pain he sustains, the type of treatment he requires, the alterations in life-style necessitated by the disease and the manner in which others view the illness and alter in their behaviour towards, and expectations for him.

Age and Level of Development
Illness causes different threats to children, dependent on their age and level of development. To appreciate this, one must first consider the nature of childhood. Essentially, childhood is a time in which the growing individual acquires all the skills necessary for separate, independent adult life. It is a phase in which the child gradually relinquishes his total dependence on others and develops a sense of self-reliance, based on his ability to explore and eventually master his environment. To fulfil his potential in this way the child needs constant opportunities and consistent encouragement to try out new skills, and continual protection from trauma which may diminish his courage and willingness to develop.

Illness, which so frequently deprives the child of freedom, a sense of independence, and the opportunities to explore and experiment, negates these strivings for self-expression, and is therefore deeply disorientating. Naturally, children of different ages, at different stages in their development, are affected in different ways.

For the infant, there are no threats in being nursed and tended

[1]For example, the life expectancy of children with cancer (Edelstyn, 1974), leukemia (Till, Hardisty and Pike, 1973) and cystic fibrosis (Dobbs, 1970) is being increasingly extended.

by another. On the contrary, this is normal for his age and essential for his survival. Serious illness should not therefore disorientate him, provided he is cared for in a familiar environment. Problems arise, however, if infants are faced with unfamiliarity, for example, if transferred from home to hospital, with consequent changes in routine. Even the youngest infants seem to respond adversely to such moves, sensing differences in handling, feeding and changing (Burton, 1975). Many become correspondingly fractious, a factor which undoubtedly impairs their powers of recovery. Such disquiet appears to stem from the disruption of the infant's secure relationship with the adult, usually his mother, upon whom he has become dependent for survival. This factor argues strongly for the extension of domiciliary care for ailing infants, and the continued establishment and use of mother and child units in hospitals.

As the young infant matures, his relationship with his mother becomes increasingly intense. He swiftly regards her as an essential source of physical comfort and also as a safe haven to which he can retreat when stressed. In addition, because she invariably encourages and provides opportunities for the gradual unfolding of his abilities, she seems crucial for the development of his skills. Illness, if it entails separation from the mother, or handling by another, is therefore a fundamental threat at many different levels. As with the infant therefore, if illness necessitates hospitalisation, every care must be taken to keep a mother and young child together. Unless the fundamental mother/child relationship can be maintained, pre-school children often exhibit protest withdrawal and despair when nursed in hospital (Robertson, 1953; Bowlby, 1971). None of these behaviours are conducive to recovery, and, if allowed to persist, may prejudice not only the child's physical growth but also his personality development both in the short and long term. Some young children seem especially vulnerable in this respect, for example, those who appear more than usually fearful prior to hospitalisation, those with few social skills, and those with no previous experience of 'happy' separations from the mother (Stacey, *et al.*, 1970; Burton, 1975).

Additionally, illness can tax pre-school children in other ways. For example, even the home-nursed child is disorientated if his need to explore and manipulate the environment is interfered with. Where he must remain cot-bound, or immobile, he may protest against the loss of his ability to walk, climb or fully participate in family life. As a result he will need compensatory provision of creative play materials, so that he can at least develop his fine skills as a counterbalance for the loss of his gross motor functions.

The ability to tend to oneself at the toilet, wash, dress, eat and drink unaided are all fundamental skills, acquired painstakingly over a period of time. None of these attributes is surrendered lightly, and children of all ages protest vehemently against yielding their control over them. This is especially true of pre-school children, whose sense of self is rooted in personal control of physical functions. Every ill child, whether at home or in hospital, should therefore be encouraged to do as much as possible for himself. This not only maintains an essential sense of independence and counteracts damaging passivity, but also gives the child the feeling that his illness is only relative, and he is still in possession of many intact faculties.

Normally, school-age children will have learned to separate from their parents, and will be used to strange environments and contacts with unfamiliar adults. If illness necessitates hospitalisation, their more developed social skills will enable them to adjust, at least if parents are able to prepare them initially for the event and accompany them during the settling-in phase. Some more fearful older children may still have problems in adapting to hospital care, however, and need special support if they are not to sustain emotional damage and associated physical decline.

One of the major problems facing seriously ill school-age children is that almost invariably illness limits the number of things they can do. This potentiates damaging boredom, and contributes to a sense of inadequacy and worthlessness. To counteract this, all seriously ill children need as rich and demanding a life as possible. Purposeful school work should never be abandoned, for school work not only fills empty hours (Oswin, 1971) but also gives the child a sense of achievement, and some hope for the future. Hospital schools, necessary even in short-stay units, are crucial in long-stay establishments and home tuition is essential for the child who is confined to the home. In addition, seriously ill children should be encouraged to be as mobile as possible, take up sports and hobbies commensurate with their physical abilities, and live each day as fully as possible.

If separation is the paramount fear of small children, pain, disfigurement, inadequacy, and ultimate unacceptibility are the essential fears of older seriously ill children. Some of these fears spring from inadequately explained—and therefore inadequately understood—treatment procedures, some from the fantasies which the child weaves concerning his illness, and some emerge from a gradual appreciation of the significance of the care which parents and hospital personnel lavish upon him. As with the fears of younger children, amelioration of these fears is essential for the older child's survival. Like the adult, he needs to know that he is acceptable to others, and that his life has value. In order to have the courage to continue he must believe there is a place for him in the world. As a consequence, children who fear personal inadequacy, often endeavour to overcome this by developing additional, compensatory skills. They frequently become more verbal, more sympathetic to others and often have a sustaining sense of humour. Some show greater fastidiousness in dress and personal appearance and, if they possess special talents, work hard to maximise these. All those surrounding the older seriously ill child should be sensitive to his fears and aspirations, and endeavour to assist him to form a realistic, but hopeful, self-image. Every child possesses some attributes which can be praised and developed.

One of the most taxing problems with older children is that inevitably, with time, most begin to sense something of the severity of their condition. As a result, some become genuinely concerned for their own mortality. Sometimes such fears are prompted by subtle changes in the behaviour of others towards them and occasionally, from the cruel taunts of other children (McCollum and Gibson, 1970). In some instances it is the death of another child in the ward, or one known through the out-patient clinic, which triggers off such fears, especially if these deaths are hastily and clumsily denied (Yudkin, 1967).

Whilst it has been known for children as young as three to voice fears of death (Wahl, 1958; Burton, 1974a), generally, their notions concerning this state are confused and sketchy, death being equated with the more fundamental age-appropriate fears of separation and abandonment. By mentioning death, very young children are usually seeking reassurance that they will not be left alone. However, children beyond the mental age of ten are quite intellectually capable of comprehending the irreversibility of death, and many are quick to deduce the severity of their own condition. Teenage patients are especially sensitive in this respect and their fears of personal extinction may become such that, in order to contain them, they are forced to deny all that is happening. Consequently, some refuse to accept the facts of their illness and repudiate any treatment procedures still available to them. Children in this state are obviously an easy prey to their disease.

Clearly, in the interests of the older child's physical and emotional well-being, gross denial of this sort cannot be allowed to persist. Whilst it is always wrong to shatter a child's own instinctive defences, with care, a relationship can be established so that the child can communicate his exact fears to a sympathetic adult. Reassurance can then be given and it is possible to reassure even a dying child. He can be assured that he will never be left alone, that he will suffer no pain and that everything possible will be done for him. More than this, such a conversation will assure him that he can honestly express whatever he feels, that his feelings will never be hastily denied or become a source of embarrassment, and that he will receive truthful answers to his questions. These assurances are necessary for children of all ages. If, in their fulfilment, we are required to extend our present domiciliary and hospital nursing care, or our present provision of effective pain control programmes, then we should make these the immediate and urgent aim of our paediatric services.

Symptoms
The previous section has emphasised the ways in which children vary in their response to their illness, according to their age and level of maturity. A child's response to his symptoms is similarly age-related.

Infants and pre-school children are essentially egotistical and rarely compare themselves with others. As a result they normally accept their symptoms, however gross, without undue upset (Debuskey, 1970). Exceptions to this rule are found, however, in families where the parents themselves are so distressed by these symptoms of their child's disease that they become acutely anxious and communicate their own anxiety directly or indirectly to the child. In such cases apprehension may be conveyed even by the mother's unwillingness to touch or handle the affected area. But, in such cases, the pre-school child who responds with anxiety is usually responding more to his parents' feelings than to actual disease manifestations. Generally, it is not until the child emerges from the age of egocentricity and starts comparing himself with well brothers and sisters, or intact schoolmates, that he develops genuine discomfort concerning his symptoms. Obviously the way in which he responds to these will largely depend upon their exact nature and the degree to which they interfere with the gradual unfolding of his abilities. Similarly, the way in which others view the symptoms will shape the child's own response to them. Where symptoms are very obvious and disfiguring, the child may respond with shame and embarrassment, especially if he is met with aversion or fear. This is especially true of children whose illness has a late onset and who have not therefore spent pre-school years accommodating to their disability. Care should be taken to constantly praise such children concerning their other intact faculties. Even grossly deformed children can accommodate to their handicap if handled with sufficient sensitivity (Oswin, 1974).

Where symptoms are less obvious, but ever present, as in the case of many chronic conditions, they may be resented because they prevent full participation in normal play or classroom activities. This both isolates the child and contributes to his growing sense of 'difference'. Parents can help in counteracting the upset this engenders by assisting the child's conformity in other ways, for example, by providing the 'right' clothes, school equipment, or hair-do.

Teenage children may worry that their symptoms will prevent them obtaining or holding down a job. These fears can be eased by parents sympathetically investigating the employment situation, or taking the child to a Youth Employment Officer, who will realistically assess the opportunities available for the child in his area.

Where symptoms are not fully understood, or emerge unexpectedly, they may produce considerable fear in parents and children. Wherever possible, both should be warned in advance of their probable occurrence. Similarly, both should be assured that nothing they did, or omitted to do, contributed to the development of such symptoms. It is not unusual for parents and children to feel vaguely responsible and even guilty for the emergence of symptoms unless proper explanations have been given.

Occasionally, parents and children assess physical progress with reference to symptoms, using them as a barometer by which to judge the child's overall physical health. Worry concerning symptoms may therefore represent worry concerning the overall illness, just as protest about symptoms, or treatment, may mask more fundamental fears. Often a child who worries or protests in such ways is expressing his fears of loneliness, difference, worth-lessness, or death, in a manner that he knows will be acceptable to others. He knows that his parents or nurses will tolerate upsets concerning symptoms or treatments and endeavour to comfort him as a result, whereas he senses, often rightly, that they may become apprehensive and withdrawn if he asks for reassurance for his fundamental fears.

Whatever the negative aspects of symptoms may be, at least they are reliable indications of disease, and children displaying them can be treated as if they are ill. In this sense their lot is easier than that of some other seriously ill children who may lack obvious or easily discernible manifestations of their condition. An apparent lack of obvious symptoms can be especially disorientating at the outset of an illness, contributing to delay in diagnosis, with consequent parental upset (Burton, 1975). Sometimes, in the early stages of a disease, ephemeral changes in the child's well-being may be misconstrued as naughtiness, and punishment may be given. Occasionally, seriously ill children have even been taken to Child Guidance Clinics for assessment and therapy before their disease has been recognised (Atkin, 1974). Such experiences undoubtedly cloud the child's attitude to his illness, and often his relationship with his parents. In turn, such experiences frequently add to the parents sense of guilt and their feelings of inadequacy to deal with the disease.

Where the disease continues without markedly obvious sympto-matology, it may be difficult for parents to really believe that it exists, and to ensure that the child receives necessary treatment. Similarly, they may encounter difficulties because the illness is taken seriously by their friends or kin. Their consequent sense of discomfort and isolation may rebound on the sick child.

Pain

Pain is not conducive to well-being at any age, yet despite this our attitudes to it are fundamentally confused (Mennie, 1974).

This is especially true of our attitudes to pain in children. Even today, many who care for young children deny that they experience such discomfort, or that such feelings are of significance in terms of their adaptation to disease. But this is not the case. Even infants show evidence of pain, although their response to it is gross, rather than discrete. With increasing age, pain becomes increasingly specific, and the child's ability to detect and report it improves. With younger children however, difficulties in management may occur because the child is unable to distinguish the area from which the pain emanates. Also he may confuse the original pain with subsequent attempts to eradicate it, and become correspondingly fractious and difficult to handle (Freud, 1952).

Older children may also become increasingly negativistic if their pain is allowed to persist. They may then respond to their illness with rage and resentment; both emotions which will prejudice their immediate physical well-being and their long-term adaptation. Children who have been mismanaged in this way may respond aggressively to even minor therapeutic procedures, trivial setbacks, or changes of environment. Similarly, parents witnessing their distress and being unable to alleviate it properly, may become equally militant and demanding.

Treatment
Many factors contribute to a sick child's willingness to accept treatment. As with his response to the illness as a whole, age and level of awareness are important considerations. So also are the nature of the treatments, the extent to which they affect his sense of physical well-being, and the attitude of his parents towards them.

Generally, children adapt best when their treatment régime is commenced in infancy and becomes part of the unvarying routine of life. Indeed, many tiny children placed on continuous medication become so punctilious about its use that they remind parents on those occasions when it is forgotten. Obviously the nature of the treatment is important in this respect; taking tablets and medicines is less disruptive of play than having postural drainage or physiotherapy. It is therefore tolerated better by children of all ages (Burton, 1975). Similarly, if care is taken from the outset to make the treatment task as pleasant as possible, it will be better accepted. Mixing tiny sweets with tablets, closing ones' eyes and counting whilst they 'magically' disappear, telling stories whilst clapping, are gambits which turn a chore into a game.

With older children, especially those diagnosed beyond infancy, treatment may be disliked because it becomes a symbol of the child's illness, accentuating his sense of difference from others. Naturally, the more obvious the therapy, the more equipment involved, the less the child can disguise it, the more embarrassing it will become. Older children therefore need careful explanations concerning the nature and usefulness of the required régime. Some parents may lack the ability to talk over such matters, either because they do not know the facts, or because they are afraid of frightening or hurting the child by voicing the subject. In such circumstances the child's own doctor may feel compelled to raise the matter, or to give the child some simple literature to read about it. In this context, voluntary societies and parents' groups could still do much to provide question and answer leaflets, specifically written for children, concerning the disease.

Some treatment procedures undoubtedly have a punitive colouring, for example, those requiring bedrest or immobilisation, swallowing unpleasant substances, or a limitation of food intake. Understandably, some children faced with such treatments see them as evidence of rejection, or view them as punishment for wrongdoing, perhaps as a dreadful adult retaliation for becoming sick. Such children need reassurance about these fears, especially concerning any sense of guilt or responsibility they may have. In extreme cases, perceptual and bodily disturbances and acute loss of identity may be found in children whose treatment demands physical isolation (Jabaley, *et al.*, 1970; Burton, 1974b). Great care must be taken to maintain verbal and emotional contact with such children and reassurance must be given that the treatment is only for their good, and that it will be discontinued as quickly as possible. Sometimes, children placed in this physical isolation misconstrue the situation, believing that they are placed apart for the sake of others, rather than for their own sake. Such thoughts should be watched for and banished before they assume frightening proportions.

One of the chief dangers inherent in home-based treatment programmes is that, occasionally, they engender an excessive sense of responsibility for the child's well-being on the part of the parents. This, in turn, tends to implicate the parents in the illness outcome and contributes to an over-zealousness on their part in administering the therapy. As a result, they may rivet on this aspect of their child's existence to the detriment of his wider social, emotional and intellectual needs. The child is thus deprived of a full existence, made more anxious for his own safety, and encouraged to become over-dependent on his parents. This in turn discourages his stirrings for independence and further diminishes the quality of his life. If at any time he becomes temporarily stronger, or more anxious, he may protest against the arrangement, repudiating the treatment. Such protests, unless properly understood, may frighten parents and child alike, alienating one from the other.

Casual observers often think that children kept on treatment for a long time must eventually adapt to it, so that in the end they completely accept it. This is rarely the case, especially when treatment procedures are unpleasant, cause discomfort, or interrupt normal life. In such circumstances children continually, and understandably, endeavour to evade them. In this context, parental attitudes are of enormous importance. Any weakness on the parents' part, or hesitation in giving therapy, is quickly recognised and exploited by the child. The child may argue that the treatment hurts, or makes him feel sick, or he is tired or fed-up. Insecure parents, unable to accept their child's hostility, or parents who have been insufficiently counselled regarding the need for such treatment, may crumble in the face of these protests. As a result, the child will probably increase his manipulations, with a consequent increase in his parents' inconsistency. Only an unremittingly positive approach to therapy will do and before this can be achieved, parents must not only be fully cognisant of how to give the therapy, but also of the reasons for its use.

The obviousness of the survival value of the treatment for the child is a further factor affecting his reaction to it. Generally, less well children respond best to therapy. Similarly, children whose treatment has markedly improved their well-being are most positive towards it.

Alterations in Life-style necessitated by the Disease
As previously stressed, infants and young children with little standard of comparison seem to adapt best to alterations in life-style necessitated by disease. By contrast, the older the child is at

the onset of his symptoms, the greater has been his previous freedom, and the harder it is for him to accept the limitations of his disease (Debuskey, 1970). Understandably, the more limiting the condition, the more exacting is this adaptation. Consequently, children with severe disabilities requiring bedrest, immobilisation, or confinement to a wheelchair often use all their self-control in maintaining a superficially accepting attitude. When additional stress is placed upon them, especially if this emanates from domestic rather than medical sources, such children frequently react with what appears, from a distance, to be excessive emotion. Simple changes in domestic routine trigger off temper tantrums; visits to the dentist prompt angry scenes; family quarrels produce disproportionate despair. It is as if the child is already so heavily burdened that he cannot tolerate any additional stress. Naturally, this makes the task of caring for such children an additionally complex one. Any change must be introduced gradually, with as much preparation or warning as possible. Parents must be advised of the need for consistency in their handling of the child, yet at the same time, they must be aided in devising a management plan which emphasises 'normality' and not damaging compensatory over-protection. It is surprising how even the most sensible parents become pamperers in the face of their sick child's protests. But pampering rarely produces any marked improvement in the child's behaviour; rather it increases his confusion and level of anxiety, and often results in growing resentment and discord on the part of his less indulged brothers and sisters.

Alterations in Parental Expectation

When parents come to realise that their child is seriously ill they frequently change in their behaviour towards, and expectations for him. Such changes emanate from feelings of concern and pity for the child, coupled with the need to avoid personal self-reproach should he die. Subtle shifts in child-rearing practices occur, most of them designed to protect the child. Thus the sick child often receives less, or no, punishment for wrongdoings, more attention in the home and less freedom to join in play or activities away from home. Protective parents frequently lower the standards they set the child in terms of school achievement and the ability to integrate well with other children. Occasionally they wish him to be less independent. Generally such changes are at marked variance from the parents' ideals of normality for the child and produce personal unhappiness and guilt on their part. These feelings are exaggerated if one parent is anxious to protect the child, whilst the other wishes to encourage him to use all his available faculties to the full. Naturally, such dissonance in parental attitude potentiates the level of anxiety in the home and affects both the sick child and his well brothers and sisters. It should also be remembered that well children are quick to notice disparities in discipline and handling between themselves and the sick child and are not impervious to consequent feelings of jealousy and resentment. Where these occur, the family is additionally stressed and the sick child is more than ever insecure and anxious.

Changes in parental behaviour towards, and expectations for, the sick child obviously influence him in different ways. If they emphasise protection at the expense of growth, they undoubtedly lessen his strivings for self-assertion, and may make him feel somehow diminished and guilty. If they over-stress the need for equality with well sibs, ignoring his physical inadequacy, they may increase his feelings of failure. If, in any way, they make him feel different from his sibs or peers, they may increase his feelings of precariousness and add to his anxiety. Disagreements between parents in terms of objectives, or animosity on the part of other children, will add to his distress. To avoid this parents should be urged to treat their sick child as normally as possible, allowances only being made for gross physical disabilities. Similarly, sick children should be encouraged to maximum achievement at a realistic level. As with well children, what the sick child must learn is 'how to capitalise on his capabilities and, at the same time, to accept his limitations' (Hewitt, 1970).

Unless such a balance can be achieved the sick child will suffer unnecessarily. Thus, damage will be done to the child which could be avoided. Frequently, when assessing the lives of seriously ill children, one is forced to the conclusion that it is not solely the illness which handicaps the sick child; rather it is the whole amalgam of improperly understood social changes, hardships and evasions which surround it. This need not be the case as is seen from the writings of many parents and clinicians (Mead, 1969; Craig, 1974). Some children not only flourish despite their illness, but are capable of showing great courage, a sustaining sense of humour, and sympathy for others.

When considering the seriously ill child's reaction to his situation it is therefore essential to remember that whilst he is uniquely stressed, so also is he offered a sterling opportunity to test the strength of the relationships which sustain him. More than any well child, the seriously ill child can be certain that he is loved, despite all his inadequacies, just for himself. As a result, feelings of closeness may develop, which enrich not only the sick child but also his parents. For this reason it is not unusual for parents to feel that they themselves have gained much in life as a result of their experiences with their seriously ill child.

REFERENCES

Atkin, M. (1974) The doomed family, in *Care of the Child Facing Death* (Ed. Burton, L.), p. 60. London: Routledge & Kegan Paul.

Bowlby, J. (1971) *Attachment and Loss*, Vol. 1. Harmondsworth: Penguin Books.

Burton, L. (1974a) *Children with Cancer*. In The Marie Curie Memorial Foundation Symposium on Cancer, the Patient and the Family (Ed. Raven, R. W.). Altrincham: John Sherratt & Son.

Burton, L. (Ed.) (1974b) *Care of the Child Facing Death*. London: Routledge & Kegan Paul.

Burton, L. (1975) *The Family Life of Sick Children*. London: Routledge & Kegan Paul.

Craig, Y. (1974) The care of our dying child, in *Care of the Child Facing Death* (Ed. Burton, L.). London: Routledge & Kegan Paul.

Debuskey, M. (Ed.) (1970) Orchestration of care, in *The Chronically Ill Child and His Family*, p. 4. Springfield, Ill: C. C. Thomas.

Dobbs, R. H. (1970) Social aspects of cystic fibrosis. *Respiration*, 27, Suppl. 196, 177.

Edelstyn, G. (1974) Personal communication.

Freud, A. (1952) The role of bodily illness in the mental life of children. *Psychoanalytic Study of the Child*, 7, 69.

Hewitt, S., Newson, J. and Newson, E. (1970) *The Family and the Handicapped Child*. London: George Allen & Unwin.

Jabaley, M. E., Hoopes, J. E., Knorr, N. J. and Myer, E. (1970) The burned child, in *The Chronically Ill Child and His Family* (Ed. Debuskey, M.). Springfield, Ill: C. C. Thomas.

McCollum, A. T. and Gibson, L. E. (1970) Family adaptation to the child with cystic fibrosis. *Journal of Pediatrics*, 77, No. 4, 571.

Mead, June (1969) *Helen's Victory*. London: The Chest and Heart Association.

Meadow, S. R. and Smithells, R. W. (1973) In *Lecture Notes on Paediatrics*, p. 249. Oxford: Blackwall.

Mennie, A. T. (1974) The child in pain, in *Care of the Child Facing Death* (Ed. Burton, L.). London: Routledge & Kegan Paul.

Oswin, Maureen (1971) *The Empty Hours*. London: Allen Lane.

Oswin, Maureen (1974) The role of education in helping the child with a potentially fatal disease, in *Care of the Child Facing Death* (Ed. Burton, L.). London: Routledge & Kegan Paul.

Robertson, J. (1953) *A two year old goes to hospital* (Film). London: Tavistock Clinic. New York: University Film Library.

Stacey, M., Dearden, R., Pill, R. and Robinson, D. (1970) *Hospitals, Children and Their Families.* London: Routledge & Kegan Paul.

Till, M. M., Hardisty, R. M. and Pike, M. C. (1973) Long survivals in acute leukaemia. *Lancet,* i, 534.

Wahl, C. W. (1958) The fear of death. *Bulletin of the Menninger Clinic,* 22, 214.

Yudkin, S. (1967) Children and Death. *Lancet,* i, 37.

3

The Seriously Ill Adult

E. WILKES

IT IS in the management of acutely and gravely ill patients that modern medicine has its everyday victories. These are so sweet and so predictable that they are not too far removed from the celluloid triumphs of popular entertainment. It is in this field that we have the opportunity to attain and use split-second diagnoses, with the arrhythmias following a myocardial infarct; for calm multidisciplinary planning under stress, as required by the multiple injuries from factory, mine or motorway; for the fusion of clinical skill with the interpretation of laboratory data, as in acute respiratory failure or diabetic coma; and for more subtle management decisions with the spinal injury or brain-damaged patient. The effective treatment of shock, the appropriate use of complex special measures and monitoring equipment, new and powerful drugs, the maintenance of the internal environment in a manner far beyond the original concepts of Claude Bernard, all stem from the admirable advances of the last quarter of a century. In this situation the doctor can be sure, scientific, and fulfilled.

But no matter how clearly we labour, sooner or later we meet the unalterable prognosis: and in our present society it is the chronic disasters of incurable illness that try us most. These form a common testing-ground for the adroit technician, the trained healer and the placebo effect: and these are our subject— forbidding and unpopular, perhaps, since for all incurable illness tries us most, at times it seems to interest us least.

When a patient of advanced years becomes gravely ill there is, of course, an infinite variety to the patterns of necessary adjustment. Some elderly patients fear death and deeply resent its imminence; but in many cases there is a background of almost physiological or spiritual fatigue, which makes possible a stoical acceptance of it. These patients are often more preoccupied by their physical disabilities—their weakness, their sleeplessness, their nausea, their incontinence, or their pain—than by the emotional turmoil of terminal illness. They may not necessarily want to know all about their problems. In every ten patients it is likely that two will know, that another three or four will have a good idea but will not discuss it frankly, and that the remaining four or five will deal with each day as it comes and rely on their nurses, doctors and relatives, to do the worrying for them. They may be accepting and uninterested, satisfied with their treatment, or stretched quietly on a rack of uncertainty. One cannot be sure.

In younger adults the situation is very often less placid and men who are dying with their professional expectations unfulfilled, or their family still vulnerable and immature, will tend to present more difficult problems of management. On the physical side they will tend to resent more than the older patient their pain and their weakness and yet, whenever these physical symptoms are reasonably helped or controlled, there will be the greater deployment of frustration, fear and resentment. Younger patients too, tend to demand more of the truth. Unlike the older, ill-educated and trusting patients, who have conditioned our senior colleagues, these patients want a more detailed prognosis from their medical advisers. In this they are sometimes failed by the natural delicacy and tact with which such a problem must be tackled. So easily this can shade off into bluster, embarrassed half-truths or professional uncertainty. Doctors rarely feel well qualified and experienced in this situation and false reassurance may offer temporary respite, but destroys trust more rapidly than any kinder attempts at sharing the unpalatable truth. Older doctors, in general, hide the truth more assiduously than their younger colleagues and the latter sometimes tell too much too soon and bitterly learn to regret this at leisure. It is advisable also, to remember with humility that even the most experienced doctor can be wrong, and that we usually know neither when the patient will die nor why. The patient who was given a prognosis of three months following laparotomy may, rarely, be alive and well ten years later. We must have the honest confidence to say that we do not know. This is often appreciated and patients and relatives hardly ever resent this. Indeed, they may gain comfort from the lack of certain tragedy among the mysteries of the future, so long as the likely outcome is not concealed.

The courage with which younger patients accept their fate when given adequate support and control of symptoms does not cease to be a source of inspiration to their doctors. It is important, however, to accept the fact that their courage has limits and will falter.

Panic and tears will take over, perhaps in the early morning, hours away from the brave ward-round face; or the truth faced fair and square can, a week later, be replaced by the feverish planning of a summer holiday that everyone knows can never happen. The doctor must also accept, and at times encourage, episodes of aggression, rejection, and resentment, and also encourage the nurses and relatives to share and endure.

These grieving episodes may be followed by a valuable era of acceptance. Often some reasonable limitation should be placed on the exhibition of grief for the sake of the others in the ward or family. Patients usually realise this and mask their feelings. They must be permitted to do this for it may be one of the last gifts they will be able to offer and from such successful self-control they will derive pride and strength.

One of the weaker areas of medical teaching is in the involvement and the leadership of relatives in routine patient care. Relatives, even if they are comparatively simple and uneducated will deal adequately with the problems of terminal illness, especially if they are warned what to expect and how to manage. What is perhaps more difficult for them than for anyone else is to see their spouse or parent slowly losing their grip, if this is accompanied by ineffective pain control, and this must always be a major preoccupation of the physician.

Between one half and two thirds of terminal patients require analgesics for effective control of pain. This pain occasionally continues for months so that potent drugs are required over long periods. On the whole, doctors are unwilling to do this, being frightened of prematurely shooting their therapeutic bolt. This fear is partly responsible for the sinister reputation of cancer and it is in most cases unnecessary. Potent analgesics given routinely, by preventing pain as well as merely treating it, can be given for months to the great majority of terminally ill patients without losing effectiveness. Good pain control can transform the morale of the patient and the atmosphere of the sick-room. However, drugs of a potency intermediate between mild analgesics such as aspirin and paracetamol and the potent opiates are being used very frequently and fairly ineffectively. Pain control is still the commonest badly managed problem in terminal illness. If the patient is in pain week after week the battle must be lost. The relatives will lack confidence and this will communicate itself to the patient, who will in turn be harassed by sleeplessness, anxiety and fear, as well as by his uncontrolled pain. There will be resentment towards the inefficient doctors and increased pressure to transfer the patient to hospital. Once there, unrealistic hopes will give way to further disappointment and disillusion.

We have learned in recent years to be less ambitious in our expectations of hospital care. After all, the buildings are old and unattractive, or modern and barrack-like. The nursing staff are overworked and consequently, nursing techniques must be carried out hurriedly. There is nothing difficult or complicated about the nursing care of most terminally ill patients, but what they do require above all else from their nurses is an atmosphere, however spurious, of leisured personal interest in their problems, while the time-consuming routines of chronic nursing care are carried out cheerfully, conscientiously and gently. This is not always attained in a busy hospital and nowhere else will they be looked after, if they are fortunate, with so much love and so much detailed knowledge as in their own home.

Despite this, dying at home is becoming less common. The age of caring relatives increases as our society ages and less than half of deaths occur at home. Because of these difficulties, special units for the care of the terminally ill are increasing, but these are an expensive way of dealing with this problem and must therefore, inevitably, remain few in numbers as centres of teaching and research, rather than as a nationwide solution to the needs of the dying patient. Care at home must remain as available and well supported as possible, and pain control is the most important single factor in maintaining satisfactory domiciliary care.

The emotional background of pain is well recognised. Vicious and intractable pain can be the presenting symptom of depression. A patient whose pain is well controlled is likely to be less anxious and demanding than the patient whose emotional and physical support is unsatisfactory. Many authorities prefer diamorphine (heroin) as the analgesic of choice in terminal illness because of its calming effect. It is possible, however, that this drug presents only marginal advantages over morphine. Good mixtures like the Diamorphine and Cocaine Elixir BPC with or without chlorpromazine are also deservedly popular.

Chlorpromazine is widely used in the treatment of confusion and as a potentiator of analgesics. It is sometimes misused in high dosage causing coma in a patient with susceptibility to premature pressure sores and inability to communicate his pain although still receiving inadequate analgesia. On the whole there is good evidence of a tendency to prescribe phenothiazines too much and morphine or diamorphine too little. Phenothiazines have a place in the management of pain especially in the elderly, but this must not be over-stated. Many respond well to simple sedatives such as diazepam.

It is tempting to use the tricyclic antidepressive drugs in cases where demoralisation is threatening, but they are usually disappointing and are far less helpful than a meaningful and helpful relationship with doctor and nurse. Occasionally, however, they do seem to work and therefore, unless contra-indications exist, they are worth a therapeutic trial for 2–3 weeks, unless side effects prove troublesome.

Anorexic patients may be chronically and mildly dehydrated, and the dry mouth associated with tricyclic antidepressives can therefore be exceptionally troublesome.

D-amphetamine is sometimes used even today in an attempt to control mood, reduce drowsiness and produce euphoria. This generally marks a therapeutic desperation on the part of the doctor and the results again are disappointing.

Steroids, of which the most frequently used is oral prednisolone although there is increasing interest in intravenous steroid therapy, certainly help to produce a non-specific feeling of well-being and diminish the general discomfort which by itself does not merit the label of 'pain', but which can prove a significant factor over a long term in the demoralisation of the patient. At times as a result of steroids the appetite is increased and nausea diminished. Pain seems to be helped by dexamethazone, not only by diminishing cerebral oedema and headaches due to cerebral tumours, but also in patients with breast cancer as specific hormone therapy.

After pain control, the high quality of the everyday care is the

B

main factor in the maintenance of morale. This presupposes, however, that the relatives are able and willing to share the burden effectively and that the housing and nursing will be of a reasonable standard appropriate to the individual needs of the patient. Ageing relatives, or relatives worried by the unknown problems of terminal illness, need respite and support or their loneliness resembles that of the patient.

General practitioner and district nurse, however dedicated, tend to under-educate and under-train relatives in the care of pressure sores, or in simple techniques of bed-changing, or basic catheter care. Incontinence is a potent factor in requests for hospital transfer and yet this can often be dealt with by fortnightly changes of an indwelling catheter in the home by the doctor or district nurse. This, however, is done surprisingly rarely. Faecal incontinence in inactive and anorexic patients taking opiates may be spurious due to faecal impaction. If malignant fistulae produce a constant seepage this may be an indication for at least inter-mittent admission to hospital.

The feeding of the gravely ill patient is something that can be easily taught. Very small helpings of everyday food and favourite dishes, preferably with good fluid and protein content, are usually much more acceptable than any invalid food. Expensive dishes and harassment of the patients to eat more by disappointed relatives are best prevented by a proper briefing.

Relatives must be warned that frequent changes of posture are necessary, but that pain-killing medication may be so timed that changes in position coincide with maximum analgesia. When the patient is reasonably comfortable and sensible, but is gravely uncomfortable on being turned, as is common with bone metastases, a gas and oxygen, or halothane, inhaler is especially suitable for this purpose and can give short-term relief.

It is important for the doctor to have occasional family conferences with those most involved with the patient, when simple points about working out shifts by relatives, prevention of pressure sores or contractures, or the possibility of the patient being able, as with strokes or cerebral tumours, to understand long after they are unable to communicate, can be discussed and amplified as necessary.

Probable complications, different ways of dying, and other problems the relatives should know about, all diminish the fear of the unknown and help the family to maintain the confidence and cheerfulness which are communicated subtly, but inevitably, to the patient. It is important also to give the patient, so much as is possible, a role to play in the household arrangements. The dying doctor may want to teach others about his condition. Others may desire to do simple work within their capacity, such as making a lampshade for the home, or a toy for the grandchildren. One of the most difficult factors in the management of the incurable is to prevent these patients being faced with responsibilities beyond their capacity. A wife who can no longer manage the house may best be moved out of it. It is equally improper to permit a premature withdrawal from the responsibilities of the everyday world. Slowly dying, underworked executives will get even more bored and bitter. The maintenance of independence by simple domiciliary-based occupational therapy or physiotherapy is easily organised and tragically deficient in our traditional facilities.

Patients are often not ennobled by suffering. Although their courage can be very often an inspiration, they can also be spoilt, trying, aggressive, or become accusing, ungrateful, confused and paranoid. These possibilities must be explained to the relatives so that they do not resent this and are not frightened too much by it.

Since the care of the patient should be unhurried but thorough, the district nurse must serve more as a teacher than is her custom. Mouth toilet, for example, is something that should be routinely delegated to relatives under supervision, and with frequent small drinks, troublesome dehydration in the terminally ill will need parenteral infusions only on the most rare and exceptional occasions.

It is very common, even in hospital wards, for patients who are terminally ill to be denied simple, but effective, palliative surgery, because the doctor has resentfully but inflexibly become adjusted to his incapacity to cure. However, many surgeons will be willing to perform procedures, such as a palliative colostomy, which will enhance the quality of the few weeks of life remaining. The removal by cryosurgery of skin or rectal tumours, especially if they are associated with ulceration, offensive smells, or tenesmus, is another valuable and helpful procedure that is not particularly distressing to those who have more than a few days to live.

To the gravely ill patient time-scales are routinely distorted and disturbed. A cat-nap of twenty minutes is thought to be a long and dreamless sleep. They become demoralised and disturbed by hours of sleeplessness and this, indeed, is one of the commonest complaints of the terminally ill who are being cared for in their own homes. Nitrazepam or chloral hydrate are probably more helpful here than the barbiturates which are so frequently prescribed; but any sleeping pill to which the patient was previously habituated should be kept on, even in increased dosage, unless it is obviously ineffective or harmful. Diazepam is a useful hypnotic and in high doses it is associated with a degree of amnesia that can be helpful. The patient eventually calmed after a major uproar and a hard fight with the nurses at 4 a.m. can blandly, after breakfast, tell all and sundry about his restful night!

Common causes of sleeplessness are pain, anxiety and wet or uncomfortable beds. These should all be corrected as effectively as possible before large doses of hypnotics are given.

Nausea and vomiting are frequent problems and none of the popular anti-emetics such as cyclizine, prochlorperazine or metoclopramide can be relied on to maintain control. However they can all prove effective in the majority of patients, especially when they can be administered by injection or suppository. Metoclopramide seems helpful especially in lesions of the upper gastrointestinal tract associated with nausea or vomiting. Chlorpromazine is also generally valuable in this connection and can be used in the absence of specific idiosyncrasy even when the patient is deeply jaundiced.

The severe cachexia of the gravely ill patient, especially if it is inexorably and gradually progressive, is not amenable to treatment although often palliated by by-pass surgery, or by excision, even partially, of the primary tumour; this in general terms is true also of the myopathies and neuropathies associated with disseminated malignant diseases.

Breathlessness is common, especially with metastases or carcinoma of the lung and these patients are often well controlled by the judicious use of diuretics, steroids and spasmolytics, if there is an element of spasm. Such dyspnoea, however, is helped more by small cautiously graduated doses of morphine or diamorphine. In view of the respiratory depression inseparable from the use of opiates, dosage should be more cautious than when used for routine analgesic purposes, and the shorter effective duration of action of diamorphine as compared with morphine is, in this particular situation, sometimes an advantage. Since anxiety is so often associated with breathlessness, reassurance, company and a tranquilliser can be of extreme value.

With bronchial carcinoma, cough can also be a troublesome symptom. Routine therapy with morphine or diamorphine often greatly diminishes distress, but additional anti-tussive therapy with heroin or methadone linctus adds greatly to good cough control. A recent survey of the major symptoms of terminal patients summarises their problems (Table 1).

TABLE I

The ten major symptoms of terminal patients
after admission (296 cases)

Pain	58%	Bedsores	15%
Incontinence	38%	Vomiting	13%
Confusion	21%	Open wounds	13%
Dyspnoea	17%	Cough	5%
Nausea	16%	Dysphagia	3%

N.B.: Symptoms such as insomnia, anorexia, depression and anxiety are excluded since, although often diagnosed, they were rarely complained of even when present, nor did they often impress the observer as a major symptom. (*Proceedings of the Royal Society of Medicine* (1974), Vol. 67, 1001–5).

Despite the importance of care for all these troublesome and common symptoms, it remains to be said again that good personal relationships and the prevention of loneliness are of paramount importance in providing high quality terminal care. In this situation the friendly and familiar priest obviously has a great deal to offer, but with many patients totally alienated from their church, ministers may be hesitant about the contribution they are able to make. On the other hand, such gravely ill patients tend to revert to the religious practices of their youth, especially if this is done in conjunction with those involved in their daily care, and tremendous consolation can be gained. But one must not be over-enthusiastic. Patients must be left as much as possible in command of their own life-style to the end, so a non-evangelical approach is appropriate and less embarrassing. The doctor, after all, has spent long years in developing technical skills and is more at home with the diagnosis of the ectopic ACTH syndrome, or the management of hypercalcaemia than with the subterfuges, grief and desolation produced by natural disease; processes crueller and more implacable even than man at his most obtuse. To deal with these we must add to our everyday equipment affection, dignity and humour to match that of our patients.

4

The Care of Older Patients

FERGUSON ANDERSON

THE AGE STRUCTURE of society is changing rapidly. Older people are everywhere in evidence; with an increasing number, especially of women, 75 years of age and over. The female outlives the male so that in many developed countries there is a 5–7 year gap between their life expectancy, and when people aged 100 years and over are surveyed, as in the Ukraine, there are seven times as many women as men (Chebotarev and Sachuk, 1964).

At the beginning of this century, infectious disease, tuberculosis and gastroenteritis were the common causes of death. Today, heart disease, cancerous diseases and diseases of the nervous system are most frequently recorded. Heart disease in old age is commonly due to coronary artery disease, cancerous diseases are predominant in the alimentary tract, and among diseases of the central nervous system the most frequent is cerebral vascular disease. Studies of the pathology of old age by Howell and Piggott (1951, 1952 and 1953) also illustrated the multiplicity of diseases in the elderly, the frequent silent onset of coronary thrombosis and the atypical presentation of some diseases.

McKeown (1965) reported autopsy findings in a series of 1,500 patients, 70 years or more at the time of death, and found disorders of the cardiovascular system coming first as a cause of death (21 per cent); second were cancerous diseases (20 per cent), and next diseases of the nervous system (12 per cent). The high prevalence of carcinoma of the stomach and large bowel contributed largely to mortality from cancerous diseases.

Of 500,000 deaths each year in the United Kingdom, half take place at over 75 years of age, over 90,000 take place at over 85, and 500 at over 100.

It has been stated that 5 per cent of people died in hospital at the beginning of the century; in contrast in 1965, 38 per cent of deaths occurred at home, and in 1970, 33·5 per cent. This may be due in part to the increasing number of solitary aged people.

Wilkes (1965) in Sheffield, demonstrated that no less than 14 per cent of patients with cancerous diseases dying at home were being cared for by relatives themselves over 70, while 74 per cent of caring relatives were over 50. In this survey, the general practitioners classed the medical attention needed by terminal cancer patients dying at home as minimal in 27 per cent, moderate in 59 per cent, and heavy in only 12 per cent of cases. Half the patients dying of cancerous diseases at home had no real nursing problems or serious suffering. Twenty per cent of patients had had real difficulties for a fortnight or less, and 15 per cent had serious trouble lasting six weeks or longer. In a survey of terminal care in cancerous diseases, Alderson (1970) found that patients were admitted to hospital in the terminal stages primarily for nursing care, i.e. because the family could not manage; only 30 per cent were admitted for medical attention.

In clinical practice in the hospital setting, women are ill for longer periods of time than men.

THE DYING

Acland (1974) defines dying patients as those in whom a diagnosis of incurable disease has been made, and whose doctors expect them to die within a few weeks or months. The common characteristic of 'the dying' as a group is the fact that their attendants expect them to die.

DIAGNOSIS

The doctor who sees previously unknown elderly patients must listen to them carefully. A diagnosis may already have been made in this particular individual and may indicate that the illness is fatal. However, while it may be true that this is the case it must not be assumed to be correct and the doctor must keep an open mind. On other occasions, the patient's symptoms may not fit into a previously experienced pattern of disease and careful thought must be given to the diagnosis. The patients have an uncanny habit of being right, and these unusual symptoms should not be classed as hysterical or imaginary.

It is essential to obtain accurate information about past illnesses and previous operations or medical treatment in each elderly person. In old age the atypical presentation of a common illness is much more frequently seen than a rare disease and in many individuals multiple pathology is found, while the onset of very serious illness may be insidious and quiet. After a careful history is taken and a full clinical examination made, bearing in mind the previously recorded facts, this may indicate that the patient is indeed dying. Care has to be taken to ensure that the complaints which the patient has are due to this fatal illness and not caused by other relatively minor pathological conditions which may make the individual's life miserable, for example, the presence of mouth ulcers or haemorrhoids. The side effects of medication with drugs, for example mental confusion or depression, and symptoms such as nausea and vomiting due to previous physical therapy, for example radiotherapy, must also be borne in mind.

At this stage it may be necessary to recommend that the older person be admitted to hospital so that the diagnosis which has been suggested may be confirmed, for it is essential to have a correct diagnosis as soon as possible. This does not mean that an elderly, weary and emaciated person, obviously in the last stages of life, should be subjected to investigation in order to satisfy scientific curiosity. On the other hand, the amazing and often unexpected ability of older people to recover indicates that where possible an accurate diagnosis must be made. It must never be assumed because the elderly individual looks so ill that in fact a fatal illness is present.

The elderly, like children, may suddenly appear desperately ill partly due to their severe reaction to dehydration and this may be caused by impairment of sensation to thirst. When fluid deprivation is restored and electrolyte balance corrected, a sudden and dramatic improvement in the general condition occurs.

After the correct diagnosis has been made, the management of dying older people involves the understanding of a complex interplay of physical, mental and social factors.

PHYSICAL FACTORS

Pain

The main problem with many dying patients and the one which causes most worry is pain, or fear of pain. Rees (1972), a family doctor, found that 44 per cent of his dying patients had continuous pain in spite of his own concern for the problem.

The care of the dying older person is somewhat brightened by the fact that pain sensation becomes less in the elderly. Rolleston (1922) thought that blunting of sensibility to pain is a beneficient process, suggesting that with gradual involution and approach to physiological death the warning normally conveyed by symptoms is no longer needed. Exton-Smith (1961) found that 13·6 per cent of elderly patients dying in a geriatric unit had pain of a moderate or severe nature. This can be compared with the Marie Curie Memorial Foundation's study (1952) where 68 per cent of a group of patients with cancer, who were of all ages, had moderate or severe suffering. Saunders (1960) in her series of 474 patients admitted to a terminal care unit found that the prevalence of severe pain was 19 per cent in patients of 70 and over and 37 per cent in patients under that age.

It is, of course, still essential to review the control of pain in older patients. The work of Saunders (1972a) has radically altered thinking about the use of the very effective pain relieving drugs available. She believes that such substances should be given regularly according to an invariable four hourly schedule. Whatever drugs are used, if pain breaks through, the dose and not the timing should be changed. Thus, once pain has been controlled, theoretically the patient should never suffer from pain again; this requires training and teaching of nursing staff. Many nurses are reluctant to give 'strong' drugs unless they feel the patient is bad enough to require them. People who are felt to be demanding, or patients with communication difficulties, such as dysphasia, may have to stress their symptoms to convince doctors and nurses of their suffering. Once the pain is overcome, then it may be that smaller doses of the pain relieving drug can be used regularly because there is no build-up and no fear to conquer.

Saunders uses oral heroin for pain relief in most of her terminal patients, including those at home, as she finds that this drug causes less nausea and drowsiness than morphine, and is more potent, while the danger of drug addiction is irrelevant in dying people. The usual dose of heroin required by mouth is 10 mg, and in Saunders' series (1972b) of 428 patients, only 19 per cent needed more than 20 mg, at any one time.

To control mild pain in the early stages, aspirin and aspirin-like derivatives may be used, and then more powerful pain relievers such as Diconal (dipipanone hydrochloride 10 mg and cyclizine hydrochloride 30 mg). This is a potent analgesic with a morphine-like action and is effective given orally. The usual interval between tablets is six hours, and as with all morphine-type drugs respiratory depression is a hazard, and caution is essential in the presence of liver or kidney disease.

Narphen (phenazocine hydrobromide) is another useful analgesic and can be given orally every 4–6 hours. It may produce a feeling of light-headedness or dizziness at the beginning of treatment, and is contra-indicated in convulsive disorders, delirium tremens, myxoedema and alcoholism. As with the previous substances, care is required in the presence of hepatic or renal diseases, and respiratory depression may also occur. Fortral (pentazocine hydrochloride) is given as a tablet at 3–4 hour intervals, after meals, and initially may produce some dizziness, nausea or headache. This preparation is contra-indicated where there is established respiratory depression, convulsive disorders or raised intracranial pressure. Narphen and Fortral should not be used if mono-amine oxidase inhibitors are being given.

Omnopon (papaveretum) is useful in moderate pain and can be used orally or by injection.

Some patients receive great relief from the Brompton Hospital 'cocktail'; one example of which is:

Morphine hydrochloride	15 mg
Cocaine hydrochloride	10 mg
Gin	4 ml
Honey	4 ml
Chloroform water to	15 ml

This mixture acts as an euphoriant as well as an analgesic. When a pain relieving suppository is required Proladone (oxycodone pectinate) 30 mg is often of use.

Daptazole (amiphenazole) may be of value in controlling tolerance to the analgesic drugs when larger doses than usual are required. It may also improve the patient's alertness and prevent him feeling sleepy all the time. Many elderly dying patients become weak and unhappy by being made too sleepy during the day and thus prevented from getting out of bed or eating, and this must be avoided if possible. Amiphenazole also controls tolerance to alcoholic drinks which are, on occasions, of immense value towards the end of life.

Drugs of the phenothiazine group often help to dissociate the patient from his illness and large doses are not required. Largactil (chlorpromazine) 25 mg, three times per day orally, may be useful, but large doses should be given with care in elderly people as the phenothiazines can cause mental confusion, or by reducing mobility can encourage the development of pressure sores.

Insomnia
The patient requires a good night's sleep, and if pain is the cause of wakefulness, pain relief may be enough to ensure this. However, it may be essential also to give a hypnotic such as chloral hydrate or one of the chloral derivatives. For older people who complain of difficulty in getting off to sleep, Heminevrin (chlormethiazole) is of use.

It is always worthwhile trying to analyse the cause of insomnia as it may be that depression, faecal impaction or a bedsore may be the real reason for the wakefulness. For depression, which potentiates pain or causes insomnia, the tricyclic anti-depressants may be of value.

More important than drugs, is the establishment of a warm relationship with the doctor or nurse. If the doctor sits down and listens to the various facets of his patient's distress, without giving the impression that he is wasting his time, and is careful to elicit even trivial-sounding complaints, pain can sometimes be relieved without resorting to drugs at all. A pathological fracture of the femur may require traction, a palliative operation may relieve distress, and radiotherapy relieves by shrinking a tumour. Hormones and cytotoxic drugs may be of value, and various neurectomies will relieve pain. Swerdlow (1973) believes that the use of chemical nerve blocking can give pain relief in even the very old and this method should not be forgotten.

The disadvantages and side effects of all these measures must be assessed against the possible benefits, and especially in elderly patients there must be clear evidence of adequate gain for the individual before any interference is considered.

In general, it must be stated that it is essential to give enough of the pain relieving drug to relieve pain. The dose of morphine, pethidine, or heroin which completely abolishes the pain is the correct dose, and if large amounts are required frequently in the last week or two of a patient's life to relieve pain, this would seem to break no rule and is an essential phase of the patient's therapy.

Nausea

Nausea is a most troublesome complaint and on occasion may be helped by the treatment of the associated depression with anti-depressant drugs, as the nausea may be associated with great anxiety.

Chlorpromazine is a specific treatment for nausea. It acts, in small doses, directly on the brain and this is part of its value when combined with opiates.

Vomiting

Intractable vomiting is one of the greatest miseries and in some patients is due to mechanical obstruction by the tumour. In others, the vomiting is associated with the drug being given and occasionally, there may be a psychological element. Opiates are reported not to cause vomiting so frequently when the patient in pain is in bed.

Anti-emetics may be used in the treatment of the vomiting, and if the first is not successful, it is worth trying different anti-emetics to find the one that suits the patient best, which may have to be given either by injection or as suppositories. Sometimes a patient will tolerate soda water or iced water and occasionally relief of pain will relieve vomiting. If persistent vomiting occurs, when the time for any form of surgical intervention is past, it may be worthwhile passing a nasal tube and instituting intermittent or continuous suction to prevent constant retching. The fluid intake can be supplemented by subcutaneous infusion with hyaluronidase, and this therapy given in order to alleviate symptoms of dry mouth and thirst, is not prolonging the patient's life unnecessarily, but is relieving uncomfortable and worrying symptoms.

Dysphagia

When dysphagia is severe, a local anaesthetic in gel form before food may be of value, and on occasions semi-solids are most useful. The patient who has had a Southey's tube passed will require watching in case this becomes blocked. When loss of appetite is the main symptom, 5 mg of prednisolone twice a day can relieve symptoms and is sometimes of use for the widespread aches and pains so frequent among many dying patients. Steroids also cause euphoria, which may itself reduce the perception of pain.

Hiccups

These are often most troublesome, being irritating and exhausting. The quickest way to overcome them is for the patient to breathe in and out of a paper bag for a few minutes. If carbon dioxide is available this can be used also as an inhalant. If the carbon dioxide fails, chlorpromazine by injection may be effective.

Cough

Persistent cough is sometimes a great worry, and a linctus like Ethnine (pholcodine linctus) in a dose of 5–10 ml, given in very hot water may help. Diamorphine is the strongest anti-tussive and may eventually have to be given by injection. It should not be forgotten that if the sputum is purulent, a short course of an appropriate antibiotic will be helpful.

Periodic re-examination of the dying patient may be unexpectedly rewarding and reveal new ways of helping the patient; for example, if there is dyspnoea, a pleural effusion may be discovered which may require aspiration. Duncan and Leonard (1965) reported radiation-induced malabsorption and stressed the importance of not ascribing every new symptom to a recurrence of neoplasm.

Tiredness

In long-standing illness there is often an increasing sense of tiredness and the use of exercise with or without physiotherapy should be considered. In the elderly, immobility may lead to stiffness and bedsores and the older patient should not be allowed to become bedridden before it is inevitable. In fact, there is much to be said for keeping the patient mobile as long as possible as this will cheer him up and help to prevent apathy, boredom and despair. Pain may prevent movement and when the pain is overcome the patient may become ambulant. If there has been an old stroke as a complication, physiotherapy for this should not be neglected, and the importance of regular chiropody should not be forgotten.

Time can hang heavily in certain phases of illness, and time to think may be a mixed blessing. It is well worth finding out if the patient has any particular ability or hobby, and every encouragement to use all his remaining faculties should be given. If the patient is able to undertake any minor work in the ward or at home this should be encouraged and praised. The help of the occupational therapist should be obtained and full use made of any facilities which are available in her department. The minister or priest at this stage may have much to offer and should be part of the therapeutic team.

The importance of adequate fluid intake, bowel regulation without discomfort and the correction of electrolyte imbalance, must be stressed in the terminal patient as in others. In dealing with all these symptoms, the doctor's enthusiasm and confidence in his therapy will be, without doubt, transmitted to the patient. While it is necessary to bear in mind that heroic measures are seldom indicated, it is also necessary to have the same interest in the patient during this stage of life as in any other. It is stressed that whether the elderly patient is nursed at home, in an institution, or by intermittent hospital admission and discharge, it is essential to make certain there is continuity of care. The elderly patient must understand clearly that during each phase of his illness his doctor knows what is happening and continues to care for him.

GENERAL NURSING

Nursing of the elderly dying patient is of fundamental importance and the mental health of the nursing staff must be kept in mind. Explanations to the nurses on each stage of care should be given by the doctor and the objective clearly stated.

In the nursing of such older patients, adequate care of the mouth is essential. It is often worthwhile re-shaping ill-fitting dentures to diminish discomfort and salivation and a constant watch must be kept for thrush. When pain relieving drugs are being used, constipation may occur and this may lead to faecal impaction, which in turn may cause retention of urine. Due regard must be paid, therefore, to maintaining a regular bowel action.

Nothing can replace good nursing in the prevention of bedsores, but ripple mattresses may be of value, while the danger of the phenothiazine derivatives causing immobility of the patient should be remembered. Good general nursing, regular turning of the patient, and adequate protein intake will help to prevent bedsores, and appropriate treatment given to redness of the skin in a pressure area. When the patient is incontinent, part of the regular nursing should be the use of a barrier cream over the affected areas whenever the bed is changed. Much argument exists on the treatment of bedsores, but prevention is far more important than waiting until the skin is broken. In early cases a local anaesthetic cream and an antibiotic powder such as Cicatrin may be of use (Lamerton, 1973).

Perhaps the most important way a doctor can help the nurse is by ensuring that while being kept free from pain the patient is not at the same time made too sleepy to eat or move about the bed; immobility is a great danger in elderly patients. When there is extreme pain on turning the patient with a bedsore in bed, Wilkes (1973) states that this can be controlled by an Entonox machine for inhalation before turning occurs. This machine delivers 50 per cent nitrous oxide and 50 per cent oxygen and enables the patient to be turned over without pain. Wilkes also believes that incontinence is not a major problem in domiciliary nursing, as sterile disposable self-retaining catheters can be used. If blockage of the tube threatens it can be washed out with a 1 in 5,000 solution of Hibitane (chlorhexidine).

Patients will often hesitate to complain about smell, perhaps in the belief that the doctor can do little about it. Wilkes found that where there is a fungating lesion in, for example, the breast, it is often possible to help by trying various hormones such as oestrogens, non-virilising androgens, steroids, progestogens, local cytotoxic drug application, or lastly, palliative radiotherapy. The local application of yoghourt to the wound quickly cuts down the smell, especially if supplemented by frequent dressings with an antibiotic impregnated gauze.

The worrying noises which may accompany the final hours of a comatose patient may be due to stertorous breathing, or the accumulation of mucus in the trachea and large bronchi. The noise due to stertorous breathing may be reduced by placing the head in the lateral position, or by using an airway to prevent obstruction of the fauces by the tongue. The frightening noise of accumulated mucus may be abolished by injecting hyoscine hydrobromide 0·4 mg, intravenously.

MENTAL STATE

It is important to remember that not only must the physical health of the patient be treated, but attention must also be paid to the mental state. Once an elderly patient has a diagnosis which indicates a fatal outcome, the physician tends to pass by this patient on the ward round; in general, people tend to turn away from dying patients. Perhaps the doctor feels his time is wasted with someone he cannot cure. He may fear that he may be asked a question that would involve him emotionally in a way for which he is not prepared, for doctors are not usually taught at medical school, or elsewhere, how to face dying patients.

REASSURANCE

In terminal illness reassurance is essential and it is often stated that people do not fear death but the process of dying. Time must be allocated by the doctor and his manner must be such that he invites questions from his patient and will become, over some little time, his patient's friend. Cramond (1970) finds that seriously ill patients consider death as a possible outcome and welcome the chance to talk about their feelings. The fact of sharing this fear with the doctor is in itself therapeutic, and promotes more confident communication between patients and doctors. Cramond emphasises, rightly, that the discussion of this fear, whether or not it is founded in reality, should be carried out only when the relationship between the doctor and the patient is sufficiently close. Both should have reached the stage where they are at ease with one another. He reminds us that the doctor is not trained to help in matters of a spiritual or theological nature and it may be that the physician should not hesitate to turn to the priest or minister for help. There should, of course, be good communication between the doctor and the chaplain, so that the latter may be sensitive to and be aware of the clinical situation in his approach to the patient.

Kubler-Ross (1970) has stated that there are five stages which most dying patients pass through. The first is that of denial and isolation, the second anger, the third bargaining, the fourth depression, and finally, there is the stage of acceptance. These different stages must be looked for and the patient should be encouraged to talk if he so desires.

Staff members caring for dying patients should receive simple training courses, so that they can comprehend what is going on; they must understand the concept of empathy. They should realise that talking to the patient will help them in talking to the relatives, and here they must realise that the relatives may feel anxious, depressed, angry or guilty themselves. Great tact, sympathy and compassion are required, and the aggressive relative must not be answered by aggression, but by explanation which may require constant repetition. At the initial stage of communication when the attempt is made to tell a near relative that the patient is dying, it seems as if the relatives were deaf and it is necessary to go over the same ground repeatedly with simple words, without using scientific jargon.

The decision to tell a patient the correct diagnosis and that he is dying is one which remains a problem for each doctor and the individual patient. This step should be taken when a close relationship has been established with the ill old person and only after careful thought. It may be easier in the elderly, as in Exton-Smith's (1961) series, one quarter of the elderly patients were aware that they were dying and most were calm and without fear.

If a decision is made that there should be a conspiracy of silence, then this must be complete and no well-meaning friend or relative, without consultation, should take it upon himself to tell the patient the whole truth with the patient unprepared, unexpecting and perhaps unwanting to receive such information. It is necessary to make sure that the lines of communication are clearly established between doctor, nurses, relatives and patient, and if the patient is admitted to hospital, between hospital consultant, nurses, family doctor, relatives and patient. If, for example, the hospital consultant writes to the family doctor telling him of some operative procedure or medical preparation being advised for the patient, giving in his letter the diagnosis, the next sentence should tell the general practitioner the state of communication. Has the patient, or the patient's nearest relative, been told the diagnosis? If so, what has been told to them, and perhaps more importantly, if they have not been told the diagnosis, what exactly has been said to them? This will save much embarrassment, loss of confidence and eventually perhaps ill-feeling between the patient and family doctor.

In our planning we must allow time for the senior doctor to interview the relatives of those who are ill and who need explanation and guidance, but he will need time also to communicate what he has said to other members of the caring team—both within hospital and without. This is an unfair burden to inflict on the most junior members of the medical staff.

SOCIAL FACTORS

Although housing of the elderly in Great Britain is gradually improving there are still many people, perhaps as many as one third of those over 65, who live alone with only outside lavatories. It must also be recalled that approximately one quarter of all people over 65 in the United Kingdom have no relatives and about the same number of people live alone. Older people thus tend to be admitted to hospitals, while the younger age groups with nearby children and reasonable housing, still tend to die at home. There is also a serious financial problem in nursing a dying patient at home. This may involve higher food bills for special diets, increased money spent on heating to keep the bedroom warm and in obtaining domestic assistance, in addition to any statutory help provided because of the difficulty of managing in unsuitable housing.

Cartwright and her colleagues (1973) found on enquiry from doctors that there were not sufficient hospital beds for some groups of patients, especially the older people who needed long-term nursing. These authors also concluded that the resources of the community service were often inadequate; nearly two thirds of district nurses interviewed felt they would like to give more time to patients with a terminal illness. Home help services also were deficient. Help at night was more often needed, as was help with incontinent patients. In this study, outside lavatories were also a problem, while washing machines, spin driers or telephones would often have been helpful in relieving the heavy burden of care. Better co-ordination of services was required.

Where should an elderly person die? From the point of view of the family it means care at home or care away. In Glasgow in 1968, 36 per cent of people died at home and 58 per cent in a hospital or nursing home. Many reasons were given for this: for example, homes which were too small; social dispersion of relatives; and the desire on the part of the relatives for a higher standard of living with a disinclination to be bothered. In fact, most people do their best to keep their elderly relatives at home when they are dying, but because they become exhausted with this work, hospitalisation may become necessary, often with deep regret from the caring relatives. For this reason, an effort should be made to involve the relatives in the patient's further care when they are in hospital. The relatives will also require reassurance, after admission has become unavoidable, by telling them what a splendid job they have done and how they could not have managed any longer to look after the patient at home. In fact, most elderly patients are admitted to hospital primarily for nursing care, because they live alone, or because the home is unsuitable.

In recent surveys it has been shown, frequently, that some co-ordinator must be found to organise the many services required to care for an old patient dying at home—the daily district nurse, night visiting, home laundry, provision of nursing aids, such as commodes, bandages, and bed linen, ways in which financial help can be given, and the arrangements made for friendly visiting if the patient is isolated. With this number of services necessary some co-ordination is essential. Otherwise, the dying patients left at home may undergo the same sort of rejection by the community as those nursed in hospital. It is suggested that this co-ordinator may be the doctor, the health visitor, or a social worker, but it is essential to make sure that all the caring services are involved, or relatives may fail to make contact with anyone, and thus struggle alone.

Gibson (1971) showed the great value and benefit of elderly patients dying in their own homes. Public reassurance is required that domiciliary services are sufficient to enable the relatives to play a full part in this care without being over-stressed.

THE USE OF GERIATRIC DEPARTMENTS

Death in the elderly may occur suddenly or be characterised by a slow decline with an aura of inevitability. Relatives are often more upset by the terminal process than elderly patients who may be confused in mind and lacking in insight. Relatives may also be suffering from a sense of guilt because they feel they have failed their elderly relations by not keeping them at home in their last illness. If dying old patients require hospital admission, this should be made simple, and should be prompt. There are some old patients who do not desire to die at home, but wish to spare their spouse or relations the worry and the trouble of a last illness, and are quite happy to enter hospital at that time. On the other hand there are relatives who greatly desire to take an old patient home for the last few days of terminal care. This means that there must be a two-way traffic and a promise of immediate re-admission given to anxious relatives who are doing their best. To ensure continuity of therapy, use can be made of five-day wards and day hospitals in the future for this type of patient.

It is likely that the trend towards dying in hospital will continue and geriatric departments must be ready for this work. All new geriatric units should have a large proportion of single rooms sited near the nursing station with excellent observation. The unit should have first-class amenity in furniture with bright colours and all modern services (Agate, 1973). If the ward sister and her nursing staff are carefully briefed and orientated towards the use of non-trained voluntary staff, near relatives can be encouraged to help with the physical aspects of nursing if they so desire, and thus feel they are playing their part. It should be possible for them to stay in hospital for some days.

THE FUTURE

Isaacs and his colleagues (1972) in a study of the terminal care of the aged in Glasgow found that the proportion of old people who died at home was little influenced by age and sex, but these two factors determined the kind of hospital facility in which death took place and the duration of hospital stay before death. A high proportion of very old patients died in geriatric or psychiatric wards rather than in general medical or surgical wards and many remained in hospital for one year or longer before dying. Indeed, females aged 85 years or over who died in hospital spent an average of thirteen months there before they died. Patients who died in medical and surgical wards, most being under the age of 75, spent an average of one month in hospital before their death. For those who died in geriatric wards the average stay was seven months, and for those who died in psychiatric wards it was no less than three years. Among those patients who died at home, few had deteriorated and died quickly. Many had been very severely disabled for weeks, months, or years, before succumbing. Almost all patients who died in hospital had suffered a period of disability at home before entering hospital and the longer their stay in hospital, the longer was the preceding period of disability at home.

Isaacs introduced the concept of dependancy, i.e. the period which preceded death at home, or final admission to hospital, during which the elderly patient suffered continuously from one or more of the following three symptoms—inability to walk without human support, incontinence, or severe mental deterioration. To this entire period of dependancy, he gave the name 'pre-death'.

Isaacs felt that older people who live alone and fall, and those with persistent incontinence, should be notified to the physician in community medicine, and that dementia must be realistically handled, bearing in mind the great strain on relatives who keep such elderly patients at home.

These suggestions could become possibilities if the services for older people are based on the health centre and the health care team. This would encourage routine visiting of those aged 70 and over by the health visitor, who could co-ordinate through the family doctor necessary services at an early stage. It is widely recognised that an expansion of domiciliary services is essential if there are to be more elderly patients dying at home, as there will be. The patient's own home and the hospital or specialised unit for the care of the dying should be regarded as complementary and those who desire and can be cared for at home should remain there, but help should be available immediately if domiciliary arrangements break down. In large cities the use of the health care team could greatly improve the conditions for old dying patients by the correct and prompt use of all the available services.

SUPPORT FOR THE BEREAVED

It is essential that immediate help is given especially to elderly people who have been bereaved. The family doctor, the clergy, the health visitor, social worker or voluntary worker all have parts to play.

Wilson (1970) studying the effect of bereavement on elderly people, as a health visitor, has suggested that this is a time when a continuing contact with a skilled visitor is of the utmost importance. The older person tends to withdraw from friends and society in general, following bereavement. Wilson considers that a most effective method of preventing social isolation and loneliness in old people is through support given at the time of greatest grief, ensuring that they do not become completely cut off from their families, friends and neighbours, encouraging the intake of an adequate diet, and that some interest is found for them. Numerous studies have shown the deleterious effects of bereavement in older peoples' mental health.

Rees and Lutkins (1967) showed a significant difference in the mortality among surviving spouses and near relatives according to whether death took place at home or in hospital. The risk of the nearest relative dying within a year of bereavement was twice as great if the first death occurred in hospital rather than at home.

EDUCATION

In general, all caring personnel should have training in the care of the dying. A random sample of family doctors were asked (Gilmore, 1974) if they had received any undergraduate education regarding the problems of the dying. The replies were that 38 (88 per cent) had none, 3 (6·7 per cent) recalled mention of this in a lecture, and 2 (4·6 per cent) remembered the subject being discussed in a clinical situation. More professorial departments of geriatric medicine are needed to teach the practice and principles of the care of old people to medical students, nurses, para-medical staff, social workers, divinity students, students of architecture and voluntary helpers. This instruction should include the special needs of those old people who are dying. Reassurance to young and old alike is required about the calm and quiet death which so many elderly people experience.

Specialised hospices or units for the dying are often centres of excellence where the methods of handling patients, relatives and voluntary workers are first-class. Such places can play an important part in the training of medical students, nurses and paramedical staff.

For medical students and doctors there is a need to make sure that our problems are not increased by prolonging a living death for elderly persons. The physician must plan each step in treatment with care, humanity and understanding for his older patient.

The consideration of each therapeutic problem must include possible side effects of drugs and keep in mind the desire of the patient to remain alert, interested and occupied. The quality of life in the remaining days or weeks must be of primary importance; age is in essence a secondary point. Hughes (1960) summarised the needs of dying patients as: companionship, a sense of security and control of physical symptoms by medical, nursing and domestic care.

REFERENCES

Acland, Sarah (1974) Personal communication.
Agate, J. N. (1973) Care of the dying in geriatric departments. *Lancet*, i, 364.
Alderson, M. R. (1970) Terminal care in malignant disease. *British Journal of Preventative and Social Medicine*, 24, 120.
Cartwright, Ann, Hockey, Lisbeth and Anderson, J. L. (1973) *Life Before Death*. London: Routledge & Kegan Paul.
Chebotarev, D. F. and Sachuk, N. N. (1964) Examination of longevous people in the U.S.S.R. *American Journal of Gerontology*, 19, 435.
Cramond, W. A. (1970) Psychotherapy of the dying patient. *British Medical Journal*, 3, 389.
Duncan, W. and Leonard, J. C. (1965) The malabsorption syndrome following radiotherapy. *Quarterly Journal of Medicine*, 34, 319.
Exton-Smith, A. N. (1961) Terminal illness in the aged. *Lancet*, ii, 305.
Gibson, R. (1971) Home care of terminal malignant disease. *Journal of the Royal College of Physicians of London*, 5, 135.
Gilmore, Anne J. J. (1974) The care and management of the dying patient in general practice. *Practitioner*, 213, 833.
Howell, T. H. and Piggott, A. P. (1951) Morbid anatomy of old age: Parts I and II. Pathological findings in the 9th and 10th decades. *Geriatrics*, 6, 85.
Howell, T. H. and Piggott, A. P. (1952) Morbid anatomy of old age: Parts III and IV. Findings in the late and earlier seventies. *Geriatrics*, 7, 137, 140.
Howell, T. H. and Piggott, A. P. (1953) Morbid anatomy of old age: Part V. Findings in later sixties. *Geriatrics*, 8, 216, 267.
Hughes, H. L. G. (1960) *Peace at the Last*. London: Calouste Gulbenkian Foundation.
Isaacs, B., Livingstone, Maureen and Neville, Yvonne (1972) *Survival of the Unfittest*. London: Routledge & Kegan Paul.

Kubler-Ross, Elizabeth (1970) *On Death and Dying.* London: Tavistock Publications.

Lamerton, R. (1973) *Care of the Dying.* London: Priory Press.

Marie Curie Memorial Foundation (1952) Report of a national survey concerning patients with cancer nursed at home. London.

McKeown, Florence (1965) *Pathology of the Aged.* London: Butterworth.

Rees, W. D. (1972) The distress of dying. *British Medical Journal*, **3**, 105.

Rees, W. D. and Lutkins, S. G. (1967) Mortality of bereavement. *British Medical Journal*, **4**, 13.

Rolleston, H. D. (1922) *Some Medical Aspects of Old Age.* London: Macmillan.

Saunders, Cicely (1960) Management of patients in the terminal stage. *Cancer*, Vol. 6 (Ed. Raven, R. W.). London: Butterworth.

Saunders, Cicely (1972a) *Care of the Dying.* Reprinted from *Nursing Times*. London: Macmillan Journals.

Saunders, Cicely (1972b) A death in the family: a professional view. In *Care of the Dying*. DHSS Reports, No. 5, p. 16. London: HMSO, 1973.

Swerdlow, M. (1973) The relief of pain in terminal illness. *Modern Geriatrics*, **3**, No. 3, 137.

Wilkes, E. (1965) Terminal cancer at home. *Lancet*, **ii**, 799.

Wilkes, E. (1973) Terminal illness at home. *Modern Geriatrics*, **3**, No. 3, 133.

Wilson, F. G. (1970) Social isolation and bereavement. *Lancet*, **ii**, 1356.

5

The Care of Patients by the Family Doctor

J. D. HARTE

INTRODUCTION

The characteristic feature of family practice is the primary and continuing care of the patient. It is this dual role which creates the problem of management of the dying patient. In primary care the family doctor will probably be the first person to become aware of the terminal nature of the illness and with continuing care he has to live with the inevitability of this knowledge. All men must die, but when they will die is not known. The doctor's medical knowledge will give him some fore-knowledge of when the death is probable. How he deals with this knowledge is the crux of the matter. What to say, when and how to speak, is a medical skill to be learned and practised.

In the normal therapeutic role the doctor seeks a 'cure' and is on the side of life. However, with the dying patient death is final and whatever the doctor does no physical cure is effective. The management of terminal care is therefore to ensure that the patient does not suffer physical discomfort, but also to see that he dies with dignity and with the minimum of disturbance to relatives. For some patients to go through the misery of their life and then to discover the truth about themselves just before they die might be an unkindness at the terminal phase of life. A man can die if he thinks that he has dealt with all the problems of his life, but if he tries to cheat himself over something, very tragic things might happen. After a death relatives may say, 'if only I could have discussed some matter with the deceased before he died but it is now too late'. How and when to make such communication is part of the management of terminal care. There is no clear rule for the family doctor; each doctor and each patient must resolve these issues within their own relationship.

For the family doctor the level of diagnosis must go deeper than that of physical symptoms. The management must be shared with many colleagues, including consultants, nurses, social workers, clergy, relatives and friends. How to deal with these various relationships is part of the doctor's skill. He must seek at all times to enable the patient to put into words what the patient feels about his fate. The doctor must discover what the patient really needs in order to face the natural course of the illness and also must help him live until he dies. If this can be done then care of the dying can be one of the most rewarding and fruitful experiences for the family doctor.

PHYSICAL NEEDS

As in any illness a basic requirement is to treat the physical needs of the patient. In terminal care, apart from therapy for specific disease, patients will have a variety of symptoms requiring treatment. In order of frequency these will include pain, sleeplessness, loss of appetite, difficulty in breathing, depression, constipation, mental confusion, vomiting, loss of bowel and bladder control and if bedridden there may be bedsores. Dr Ann Cartwright in *The Study of Needs of the Dying Patient* found that a distressingly high proportion of people with such symptoms had not sought help from their doctor. Some had had symptoms for over a year and tended to accept them with discomfort and resignation as part of the condition. It is valuable for the family doctor to have a check list of such symptoms and actively ask the patient about them. Their relief should be the physical therapeutic objective of each visit.

In most studies concerning terminal care pain is said to be the commonest disturbing symptom requiring relief.

Difficulty with breathing, depression and sleeplessness are the most persistent symptoms. The younger patients are most likely to suffer from vomiting and pain and the older ones from incontinence and mental confusion.

A time is reached when active treatment ends and the therapeutic objective is to maintain as much comfort as possible. Dr Cicely Saunders (1967) has contributed greatly to the knowledge of the control of pain and distress in terminal illness and emphasises the importance of a complete history and analysis of the symptoms. Each doctor will have his own way of dealing with these common symptoms, but such treatment is so often omitted that it needs emphasising. When drug administration is well managed in terminal illness there is rarely any need for large doses at any one time. Small frequent doses of analgesics and drugs influencing mood will usually make it unnecessary for heavy sedation. Patients do not like the affects after sedation. The aim should be the full relief of the symptoms but to leave the patient with the capacity to be as active as possible and able to enjoy communication with relatives and friends. If heavier sedation is necessary, before it is given, the emotional needs of the patient must be fully assessed and any underlying anxiety discussed.

Many doctors feel they can adequately deal with their patients' physical condition at home, where normal family relationships can be maintained. However, there are limits to the ability of the family to deal with the stress of caring for a dying relative, and the family doctor must be sensitive to this and may find this an indication for hospital admission. He can still, however, continue to visit the patient in hospital and keep in touch with the relatives. It may not be possible to relieve intractable pain at home and the patient may need intermittent admissions to hospital. There are a limited number of hospitals, such as St Christopher's Hospice, which provide specialist treatment of terminal care. Many family doctors would welcome direct access to National Health Service beds which they could use for terminally ill patients and so retain full responsibility of the treatment, but at present a patient usually has to go into a bed in the local district hospital.

For details of specific drug therapy the reader is referred to Chapter 13.

THE FEELINGS OF THE PATIENT AND THE DOCTOR

The family doctor needs to discover what the patient feels about his illness. Initially, the patient may not fear death, but sooner or later in terminal illness the patient begins to wonder why he is not getting better. He considers death as a possible outcome and although he may not ask directly, he may search indirectly for confirmation of his fears. He has already guessed or half-guessed the truth and depends on the doctor to give him the confirmation in an acceptable manner. Frequently, this is achieved by non-verbal communication, or in some other way, such as discussing the death of a favourite animal who really represents the patient himself.

Some patients fear death, but more often there is a fear of the process of dying. Will there be pain? Can they bear it? Will they be abandoned? Will they break down? There is often a silent grieving especially in the younger patient with unachieved aims. Feelings may develop into anger and depression and this may be dealt with by denial, withdrawal, or sometimes excessive euphoria. The emotion can be a mixture of hate and love and can be transferred to the doctor or others caring for the patient. Such feelings will often appear at the same time and unless identified and understood by the doctor, he can easily find himself reacting against them. This accounts for some of the disturbing emotional situations which may culminate in the transfer of the patient to hospital.

The family doctor is in a good position both to understand and meet the patient's emotional needs. He has some idea how the patient has reacted to previous illnesses, and what sort of relationship he has with the family and with the doctor. We tend to die as we have lived and the diagnosis of the overall life situation is the first step which the doctor has to take in predicting how the patient will react to death. The patient who fights must be helped to fight, although both doctor and patient may know that defeat is certain. The complaining type of patient will complain and the doctor must accept these complaints. The patient must be considered as a person and not the bearer of a fatal disease. The patient who delays reporting symptoms to the doctor is demonstrating anxiety about his illness. Kubler-Ross (1969) has eloquently described the emotional feelings of patients and their relatives and makes a plea that the feelings, wishes and opinions of the patient should be heard by the doctor.

MANAGEMENT OF THE DYING PATIENT

How then does the doctor proceed? Should he enquire, or be kind and attentive and ask no questions? How much can the doctor get involved in the very deep feelings of the terminal care of patients?

In a recent Balint seminar which studied these relationships and followed 120 cases over four years it became clear that if the doctor and patient could talk about the impending death, anxiety was diminished. If the knowledge that the patient is dying is, however, kept secret and the doctor pretends there is nothing wrong, anxiety increases. It is only when a patient cannot understand how he feels about illness that he seeks help. If he does not feel well, is lost and frightened, the chief problem which he cannot solve without help is the nature of his illness. What is it that causes his pains and fatigue and frightens him? If after a series of careful examinations the patient is told there is nothing wrong, and yet still feels ill and unable to understand his pains and fears, he feels let down. The doctor wonders why the patient is edgy, aggressive and resentful and why he has not been able to reassure him. If, on the other hand, the patient is given a label such as pneumonia, or an ulcer and still does not improve, this little knowledge without medical understanding can also become terrifying. It is therefore necessary to have an overall diagnosis of the whole patient and recognise emotional interactions in the total management. If the patient does not appear to be reassured then this needs to be discussed with him and understood.

Whether the doctor should tell or not is irrelevant. The doctor certainly should not lie, but equally should not force the truth on a reluctant patient. He must listen and understand, be sensitive to indirect questions and allusions, and understand the covert as well as the overt communication. The doctor should answer truthfully as much as the patient wants to know and never set out to deceive. What is important is how the doctor shares his knowledge of the illness with the patient. This is a special skill and in doing this the message about impending death can be disturbing and depends as much upon the recipient as upon the message itself. How does the doctor know that the message can be trusted to the patient and that the doctor can trust himself to manage the situation once the secret is shared with the patient? The best reassurance is certainly not promises. Usually, the patient must lead and the doctor follows.

The doctor must examine his own attitude towards death so that he can talk without anxiety and listen and look for cues as to how the patient feels and reacts. Those doctors who have a need for denial themselves will find it in their patients, and those who can themselves talk about terminal illness will find that the patients are better able to face and acknowledge it.

Malignancy and death are often associated, so that cancer creates a feeling of impending doom. This is not by any means so and patients' attitudes to malignancy must be understood. A patient who asks 'Do I have cancer?' can be answered by saying, 'If so, what does it mean to you?' Similarly, a point blank question, 'Am I going to die?' can be answered, 'Tell me what this means to you.' As a preliminary response this will reveal the patient's feelings and so enable the doctor to plan the next question and answer. A patient with cancer need only be considered as having a terminal illness when the disease progresses and the patient reaches the stage where he begins to realise that he is not going to get better, and his general condition is deteriorating. In communication with the doctor some patients make it easy, as illustrated in the following case record.

Case 1

Mr F, aged 76, a widower, a kind and reasonable man with morals and religious beliefs, was a former soldier with a military medal. His wife died of cancer. His own illness came on suddenly with very similar symptoms to those of his wife. He had a laparotomy and told his doctor that he knew the operation had not been a success. Was it something nasty? To this the doctor answered, 'Yes, you know it is a growth; now we have cleared the air we can talk about how we are going to look after you.' Following this, the patient and his family were greatly relieved and until the patient died he talked a great deal with his doctor about his ambitions and his frustrations, but was not willing to talk about his family. He showed no fear or withdrawal from the doctor on having shared the truth with him and the doctor became his trusted friend. The doctor did not tell the patient but allowed him to ask. He encouraged the patient and promised to stay with him. The doctor sensed that the patient could be trusted because he had made an overall diagnosis of the life situation. This was a soldier who had been on difficult missions, was awarded a military medal, a man who could face up to boxing and rowing and had strong religious beliefs. Once there had been an honest discussion, tension and anxiety were reduced, mutual trust developed between doctor and patient and it was easier for both to accept that death was coming.

All patients are not so accommodating and often it is not easy to trust the patient, or to arrive at a diagnosis of the life situation. It is possible under these circumstances for a 'conspiracy situation' to develop, where different persons, frequently relatives or other doctors, seek to withhold the fatal diagnosis from the patient. The conspiracy results in strained relationships in all and the doctor must always take care never to be involved. The conspiracy arises when two other people agree not to discuss the situation with the dying patient. If the family doctor discovers there is a conspiracy then he must seek to understand how it started and find out its implications. It more often occurs where there has been an inadequate life situation, or a doctor finds himself caught by his own promises as illustrated in the following case record.

Case 2

Mr F, aged 55, had an inoperable cancer. He was a well-built man but suddenly began to lose weight and experience indigestion. He was thoroughly investigated and was found at laparotomy to have extensive metastases. The patient's wife was told the truth and immediately asked the doctor not to tell her husband and he agreed. The doctor was tied by his promise and also by his own dislike of the thought of death. Ultimately when the patient was very near the end he asked straight out, 'Have I got cancer, am I going to die?' The doctor answered, 'Why do you want to know?' and the patient replied, 'Well, if you tell me I have cancer and it is fatal then I will accept it and prepare myself to die, but if you say there is a chance, there will be some hope.' The doctor again told the patient that he might get better and felt that he could not follow any other course.

The situation was more poignant since in the light of developments there were indications that the patient could have had more peace if he had known the truth. If a couple have shared their lives with the good and bad things together then surely, their greatest trial, the death of one and the bereavement of the other must also be shared or it becomes more bitter. It may be the family doctor's privilege to help them through this crisis by support and encouragement and by helping them to communicate with each other even in the shadow of terminal illness. Where one partner specifically requests that the other should not be told the truth, it will repay to discuss what this means to the person making the request and to examine the marriage relationship.

Not infrequently a hospital surgeon may tie the family doctor's hands by reassuring the patient that all has been done, though he follows it up with a letter to the doctor with the real diagnosis and may comment, 'I have, of course, not told the patient that he has cancer.' An air of optimism and reassurance may initially help the patient, but as soon as his condition deteriorates then the general practitioner need not be tied, but before speaking further with the patient should discuss the matter with his colleagues. Certainly, much misunderstanding could be avoided if doctors would communicate with one another about the patient's feelings and share their knowledge of what has been said. When a relative asks that the patient should not be told, cannot the doctor answer, 'Look, will you leave it to me? I shall bear in mind what you tell me but you must realise that there are very important other problems at stake. You must trust me that I shall try to do the right thing.'

The right thing will depend on the patient. To rush and force upon the patient information which he does not want, or is not prepared to accept could be just as devastating as not allowing the patient to speak.

THE PRE- AND POST-ACKNOWLEDGEMENT PHASE

There are two phases of communication in respect of the dying patient. The first is pre-acknowledgement and the second post-acknowledgement. The awareness of impending death may be gradually recognised by both patient and doctor. Eventually the time comes when patient and doctor acknowledge their mutual awareness. This need not be verbal and may consist of a tacit understanding that the patient understands that the doctor knows that the patient knows. It is the acknowledgement that matters and its effectiveness will depend on the quality of the doctor/patient relationship. It is important that in the pre-acknowledgement phase the doctor should work very hard to improve his relationship with the patient. This often means paying frequent visits to the patient, with informal talks about the family interests

c

and hobbies. This is not pastoral care. The doctor is sensitive to every communication and is listening to what the patient is trying to say about himself. This is a vital part of the family doctor's skill, as illustrated in the following case record.

Case 3

Mr K, aged 56, an engineer, married with one son, had cancer of the urinary bladder. He had known the diagnosis for five years and had remained at work until his condition deteriorated and he found it too much of an effort. He asked if the growth was extending and the doctor said, 'What does that mean to you?' His reply was, 'Perhaps it is that I am not going to get better.' The doctor said 'Yes' and reassured him that he would continue to help and would continue seeing the patient. He visited the patient weekly and found the relationship strained and angry. On one day he stayed longer with the patient and invited him to discuss why he felt so angry. The patient replied that the doctor when he visited gave him a prescription, did everything right, stayed for ten minutes and then left. The patient was made angry because the doctor was well enough to go about his work, while he could no longer do so. The doctor shared this sadness with him and the patient then said that he enjoyed the visit of the local priest who also visited him weekly. When asked what happened he said that the priest talked about football. The doctor took the cue and talked about the garden and during the remaining weeks of the patient's life, discussed the whole of his impending death in terms of the garden; how some of the flowers would not come up next spring. A warm relationship developed, the patient made his will, put his affairs in order and had a peaceful death. Afterwards it was found that he had stopped taking his tablets, had spoken to his wife about his death and she had a much easier bereavement than had been expected.

The doctor had treated the patient as a living person. He did not write him off, but was willing to give time and extra visits as part of the price that had to be paid. In this way the pain of dying had been lessened and frequently, if this is done drugs can be abandoned or reduced. This is illustrated again in another case record.

Case 4

Mrs W, aged 69, was a small, plump, cheerful and wrinkled-looking woman, who had abdominal discomfort for several years. She suddenly lost weight, became anaemic and had gastric bleeding. Investigations and a laparotomy disclosed an inoperable cancer of the bowel. She had never been very forthcoming about her past history. She had been married twice and her first husband had died fifteen years before. She and her husband were always very friendly, but there seemed to be underlying tensions which could not be discussed. After her discharge from hospital she had a fistula and had to be re-admitted for a further period. Following the second discharge she acted as if she would deny the illness, but her eyes contradicted this. The doctor, noticing, said, 'I see in your eyes that you are trying to ask me something but cannot say it. Can we try together to see what it is?' She answered, 'I am sure I'm all right but I don't feel I am going to get better. I think I have had an ulcer removed.' Then after a pause she added, 'The surgeon said I had a malignant growth.' After a further pause she asked, 'Have I got cancer?' The doctor, realising from her eyes that she already knew, answered 'Yes', and she said, 'I am pleased to know.' She wanted to live and despite the discharging fistula she went on holiday and gradually, over a period of time, talked about herself and her past. She moved from a country cottage into a modern flat in the town and despite apparent denial was gradually putting her affairs in order. There was gradual deterioration and she developed faecal vomiting and subacute intestinal obstruction. She complained of abdominal pain and was given opiates, needing a nightly injection of morphine. After ten days the doctor felt that there was more than physical pain and he forgot to give her the evening injection. He realised the significance of this and discussed it with her the following day and his own feelings about the omission and said, 'I did not come to see you last night. I have been unhappy about giving you morphine. I feel that perhaps there are some other things we have not yet talked about.' She sat up and said, 'I don't want to be disturbed very much.' The doctor responded, 'I don't want you to say anything you don't want to, but I am willing to listen.' She then poured out her feelings about her first marriage and how she and her present husband were lovers before her first husband had died. It was clear that for a long time she had wanted to talk about this. In the middle of talking she sat up and said it was very difficult to get her breath and her first husband had died of asthma. She seemed to be quite aware what the other pains were and was very pleased to talk when she knew the doctor would listen. That night she slept soundly without any morphine and needed no more morphine until she died about a week later.

In the post-acknowledgement phase a number of patients will acknowledge their impending death, but then appear to ignore the situation and live out a charade as if nothing was going to happen. This is exemplified by the following case record.

Case 5

L.G, female aged 62, had married a man 40 years older than herself, and been a widow for many years. She had a boarding house for students. Cancer of the breast was diagnosed two years before. She seldom saw the doctor. At the first visit she said, 'I will rest and I will be all right in about four months.' She went on as if nothing had happened. Later when the disease became more extensive she was admitted to hospital and the doctor spoke to her in more detail. She laughed and said, 'You are trying to tell me I am dying aren't you?' When he answered 'Yes', she said, 'I knew you knew I knew.' From then on the atmosphere cleared, but it made no difference so far as she was concerned and she went on acting as if she would live for a long time and there seemed to be no reason why she should not play it this way.

In patients dying from cardiac conditions there is frequently less tension. The doctor usually feels there is something that he can do and is more at ease. Patients in cardiac failure and awaiting cardiac surgery often show a remarkable lack of fear, even if they know an operation might be fatal. They prefer the chance of a better life, or death, to cardiac invalidism and often have enormous faith in the medical profession for a chance of cure.

In the post-acknowledgement stage the patient may ask questions the doctor cannot answer. It may be of value to give the patient an opportunity to discuss spiritual matters and with the patient's agreement there is usually no difficulty in turning to the minister or priest for help. It is important that the doctor should not hand over to another person, but share in the involvement to avoid the fear by the patient of being abandoned. It is also important that the patient should know that the doctor has communicated with other professional people who are involved to ensure a good relationship between all concerned.

CONCLUSION

The management of terminal illness by the family doctor is in the exploration and development of the doctor/patient relationship where the feelings of patient and doctor are fully expressed and understood. A good relationship is best established when the patient and doctor acknowledge, either overtly or covertly, their awareness of impending death and the patient is allowed to test out the relationship without any fear of the doctor withdrawing. The patient must be allowed to say what it means to him not getting better. If he says, 'I am going to die,' to be allowed to be asked what this means and then to be lead gently along to discuss his own feelings about his life, so that he can then be given some of the truth as he demands it. The doctor must always listen, stay with him to the end and be willing to share in the pain of the separation. This is what family medicine is all about, to serve life and not death in an ongoing relationship with the patient.

ACKNOWLEDGEMENT

This paper is based upon a five year research project on the doctor/patient relationship and the dying patient in Dr M. Balint's Wednesday General Practitioners seminars. Acknowledgement is made to Doctors Green, Holland, Hodgson, Hunt, Tunnadine, Lisyak, Ratoff, Marinker, Ball, Trent, Fraser, Graham, and Mrs Sandler, Mrs Bloomfield, Mr Woodcock, the late Dr M. Balint and Dr Lasman.

REFERENCES

Balint, M. (1957) *The Doctor, His Patient and the Illness.* London: Pitman Medical.
Balint, M. (1957) *Problems of Human Pleasure and Behaviour.* London: Hogarth Press.

Balint, M. (1972) Transcripts from Balint Seminars, 1966–1972.

Beattie, J. (1964) *The Doctor, the Patient and the Art of Dying*. London: Christian Medical Fellowship.

Cartwright, Ann, Hockey, Lisbeth and Anderson, J. L. (1973) *Life Before Death*. London: Routledge & Kegan Paul.

Cramond, W. A. (1970) Psychotherapy of the dying patient. *British Medical Journal*, **3**, 389.

Felgenberg, L. (1972) *Humane Death*. Personal communication.

Gavey, C. J. (1952) *Management of the Hopeless Case*. London: H. K. Lewis.

Glaser, B. C. and Strauss, A. L. (1966) *Awareness of Dying*. London: Weidenfeld & Nicolson.

Harte, J. D. (1974) *Treatment of Chronic Pain*. Lancaster: Medical & Technical Publishing Co.

Hinton, J. (1967) *Dying*. Harmondsworth: Penguin Books.

Hopkins, P. (Ed.) (1970) *Patient Centred Medicine*. London: Regional Doctor Publications.

Kubler-Ross, Elizabeth (1970) *On Death and Dying*. London: Tavistock Publications.

Lewis, C. S. (1961) *A Grief Observed*. London: Faber & Faber.

London Medical Group (1970) *Matters of Life and Death* (Ed. Shotter, E. F.). London: Darton, Longman & Todd.

Parkes, C. M. (1972) *Bereavement*. London: Tavistock Publications.

Pearson, L. (1970) *Death and Dying*. Cleveland, Ohio: The Press of Case Western Reserve University.

Pelgrin, M. (1961) *And a Time to Die*. London: Routledge & Kegan Paul.

Saunders, Cicely (1967) *The Management of Terminal Illness*. London: Hospital Medicine Publishers.

Toynbee, A. *et al.* (1968) *Man's Concern with Death*. London: Hodder & Stoughton.

6

Nursing the Dying at Home

ESME FEW

To every thing there is a season, and a time to every purpose under the heaven: A time to be born, and a time to die

Eccles. 3: 1–2

A PLACE TO DIE

It has been said that Western man living in a twentieth century civilised society has abdicated his right to choose the place where he is to die. It is, perhaps, well to remember that within this same society a great fear of dying is also held by the majority. Doctors and nurses are no exceptions and can not only implant their own feelings and attitudes upon the friends and relatives of their patients, whilst keeping a conspiracy of silence with the patient himself, but can also mask real feelings of sympathy and compassion for the sufferings of others, beneath brusqueness of manner and platitudes. It surely cannot be wrong to fail sometimes in medical, surgical and nursing techniques against the heavy odds of incurable disease, severe injuries and known malignancy. Real failure in these circumstances, lies in the inability to give time, compassion and skill to the patient who happens to be dying and to his friends and relatives.

This philosophy makes a personal demand on every professional man and woman. The personal contract which commits the doctor to care for his patient is brought into sharp focus when that care means attending a dying patient in his home with bewildered and grieving relatives. There are no neat and sterile wards with the accompanying barriers of delegated care to medical and nursing ward teams; just the realities of compassion and trust. It is here, too, that community nursing comes face to face with the real dedication to service which is the basic quality of the nursing profession. It also commands the improvement of the present traditional patterns of the transfer of patient care between hospital or specialist care and community, or generalist care.

In hospital, the dying patient should receive every attention, constant medical and nursing care, the advantages of modern palliatives, properly planned drug administration for the control of pain and freedom from neglect or loneliness. He may sometimes not be able to enjoy the uninhibited affection of his whole family. At home, some opposites can apply. Medical and nursing care is of the visiting variety, modern palliatives and proper drug régimes are frequently poorly administered, friends and relatives must become closely involved in the care required and neglect, when it occurs, is therefore from lack of professional knowledge. Loneliness and isolation from all members of the family need not happen, except when the loneliness comes from within the spirit and when there are no friends or relatives to care for the dying patient living alone.

Very little work has been done to estimate the numbers of patients who die at home compared with those who die in hospital. Ninety per cent of all episodes requiring medical and nursing attention are dealt with in the community, but it is unlikely that a similar percentage rate applies to death. Even so, when terminal illness is diagnosed, consultation between all concerned should determine the future pattern of care. This in effect means team discussion between the hospital-based medical and nursing specialists, the primary care team which is community-based, the patients' relatives or friends and, when appropriate, the patient himself. So much will depend on the prognosis, the technical apparatus required, the suitability of the family home versus the hospital ward and the availability of proper support services.

It is perhaps worth highlighting the problems which can arise from poor communications in the case of the patient who is going in and out of hospital. In an integrated service there is no excuse for failing to appreciate that on-going care is all the better for co-operation and planning, rather than crisis decisions to send patients home at short notice. Decisions to transfer patients ought to be made in their best interests, rather than in response to the urgent demand for an empty bed, however pressing that may be. If someone is ill and needs attention then, hopefully, more effective communications between nursing staff will develop. It is particularly trying to the primary care team if ill patients are sent home at weekends without prior consultation. The health visitor or district nursing sister should supply comprehensive reports on the care given at home as the patient passes into the care of the ward-based nursing team and vice versa.

Once the decision is made, the transfer from hospital to home care should be effectively planned, so that the home, family and the primary care doctors and nurses are all prepared. This requires good communication systems and the transfer of the correct facts about diagnosis, prognosis and treatment between professionals. Even if it is not the appropriate time for the patient to know the true nature of his illness, the family must know. These details may need to be re-told by the family doctor, for in the stressful situation of the hospital setting, it must be recognised that people do not always fully comprehend what is said to them.

There seems to be a great reluctance and anxiety by relatives to look after dying patients at home. This could largely be explained because they do not know what to expect and their fears of death and feelings of helplessness, together with distress, inhibit their courage and capabilities. If doctors and nurses adequately discuss with the relatives, the pattern of the disease, life expectancy, treatment and care and exactly how the patient's last few days will be spent, then the problem will be largely resolved. The burden will seem less awesome and, secure in the knowledge that they will have medical and nursing support, relatives can participate in a major caring role.

THE TEAM TO CARE

In recent years there has been considerable improvement in the understanding of the extents and limitations of home care. This has been largely brought about by the attachment of home nursing sisters and health visitors to general practice and by the activities of the general practitioners themselves to advance training for doctors in general practice. Community nurses also have demonstrated increasingly to their hospital colleagues the pattern of their work and the range of their case loads. Collectively, these have interacted to provide a sound basis for a team approach, comparable to the ward situation, of doctors and nurses working together to maintain their patients' health or to sustain, treat and rehabilitate them in disease.

The health visitor, male or female, is a State Registered Nurse with obstetric experience who has also acquired the Health Visitor's Certificate. The home nursing sister is a State Registered Nurse, male or female, who may well hold additional qualifications and has normally taken the training required to achieve the National District Nursing Certificate. The Joint Board of Clinical Nursing Studies has prepared an outline curriculum in the Care of the Dying Patient and His Family. The aim of this course is to train nurses to the highest professional standard in all aspects of care of the dying, to give patients the best quality of life during their last days and help them to die with dignity, in comfort and tranquility.

It is hoped that many nurses in the community will be enabled to take such additional training so that they may better assist their doctor colleagues to provide high standards of care to the patient dying at home. The confidence of the hospital medical and nursing team in the adequacy of care provided by the primary care team should thereby be ensured. But the opportunity to meet together to exchange professional views would be of great advantage.

Other members vital to the caring team will be State Enrolled Nurses, working with the Home Nursing Sisters, who may also hold a National District Nursing Certificate, and Nursing Auxiliaries. These nursing staff give much sound basic nursing care and comfort to their patients and the families they visit. Finally, the contribution of relatives and friends is vital, since the district nursing service can only be provided on a visiting basis. The nurses therefore teach the relatives essential nursing tasks such as care of the pressure areas and care of the mouth. They can then confidently help their sick relative.

Occasionally, the community nurses will be involved in the basic education and training of student nurses. With the present syllabus more student nurses are spending several weeks in the community field and are able to participate in the team care of the terminally ill. Some of them find the experience unique in the whole of their training. To quote one example, a student nurse was able to support an early teenager through the agonising period of losing her mother from carcinoma and witnessed the devotion of the husband in caring for his dying wife. The introduction of a student to the home nursing situation, however, places additional responsibilities upon the nursing sister concerned and must never be allowed to disrupt the nurse/patient/family relationship which has to be carefully built up. It is rewarding to note that more medical students are taking the opportunity to visit patients in their own homes with the community nurses.

THE NATURE OF THE DISEASE

No dissertation on the care of dying patients should exclude a comment on long-term, incurable, or progressive illness. Community nurses are familiar with dealing with conditions such as multiple sclerosis and post-cerebal vascular accident as well as malignant diseases. Deterioration in health over one or more years requires as much planned care as short-term, more dramatic, terminal care.

It has been said many times that modern medicine has become adept at preserving life in quantity, but in the community a major concern is to ensure, as far as possible, the quality of that life. It is difficult to nurse the unconscious patient other than in hospital, unless the cause is coma prior to death. Yet an elderly woman can live alone at home, suffering from progressive disease, chair-ridden, whose only regular daily contacts are the home help and district nursing sister.

Rehabilitation is, in general, poorly practised and should mean an endeavour to assist the patient to achieve the maximum standard of life potential of which he is capable. This will require a variety of services, including speech therapy and physiotherapy, to be made available at home. At present, community nurses undertake much of the rehabilitative programme and expanded services into the community are much needed.

Many patients are assessed in the hospital situation and enjoy concentrated rehabilitative treatment. When no further progress can be made and they return home, a certain standard of continued care should be provided. This demonstrates, yet again, the communication links that must improve between specialist teams in hospital and generalist teams in the community. The provision of day care units should also be increased.

The responsibilities of Social Services Departments within the local authorities, concerning the provisions of the Chronically Sick and Disabled Persons Act, 1970, should make help available for both long and short-term conditions and social workers should become valued colleagues within the primary care team. The collaboration machinery, implemented as a result of the re-organisation of the National Health Service, should examine the provision of support services in respect of long and short-term terminal illness.

The nature of the disease determines the type of demands made upon services and skills. Because some patients are a longer time dying than others, the demands are often greater and extended over long periods of time. Loneliness and fears may be more acute as well as exhaustion of relatives and friends. Community nurses can sometimes arrange for patient care in hospital or a welfare home in order that devoted relatives may have a holiday. Night sitter services, where provided by Social Services Departments, offer a night's rest to the family. But courage is much needed, many persons strive for high ideals and everywhere life is full of heroism; those who care for the terminally ill at home should be ever mindful of the stresses and strains of the family under these circumstances.

PRACTICAL CARE

The competence of the well qualified nursing team in the community has been established. Ideally, the home nursing sister or the health visitor will have been involved in the planning required before the dying patient is returned home. The relatives should have been seen at home and the most suitable preparations made for the sick room.

Equipment is usually best ordered in advance by the nurses, in consultation with social work or occupational therapy colleagues. This will avoid the duplication of orders which sometimes occurs and also ensure the practical advice of the nurse who will know what she requires for the comfort of the patient and her own efficiency. Most Area Health Authorities will have a medical equipment loan service and there is usually a wide range of equipment available, examples being ripple beds, hoists, sheep skins and commodes. Adaptations to the home can be arranged through Social Services Departments and aids to daily living provided. The nursing sister will, of course, have instruments for dressings and other treatments, but there is still not enough provision made for the use of central sterile supply packs by community nurses.

It is helpful if a small supply of drugs and dressings or other special requirements of the patient can be provided by the hospital upon the transfer home. Considerable difficulties have been experienced when patients are sent home without supplies, particularly at the weekends. Thereafter, supplies are prescribed by the general practitioner on E.C.10 forms.

Incontinence is as distressing at home as in the hospital ward. The family is required to maintain continual supplies of clean bed linen and any ward sister will appreciate what a difficult task this must be. Home nursing sisters can provide incontinence pads and special polythene sheeting can be used to protect mattresses. Some local authority Social Services Departments provide limited soiled laundry services but, generally, the family bears the brunt of the problem. It must be remembered too that elderly patients living on a pension can afford only a limited supply of bedding. In a comprehensive health service designed to meet the health needs of people, this is an area that might qualify for a central supply and access to laundry services in future. The control of malodorous material is often difficult, and effective aerosols and deodorising agents are necessary equipment for the home nurse.

When the patient can get up for washing and visits to the lavatory it is easily recognised that it can be less stressful for him to walk across the landing to the bathroom than the length of the ward. It is different if the lavatory is shared and one floor down in a tenement block. The provision of commodes has already been mentioned and bedpans and urinals are also obtainable. They do, of course, require emptying and cleaning, tasks frequently shared with the family by the community nurses.

The disposal of soiled dressings and nursing debris is mentioned. Disposing of disposable equipment creates its own problems. Items such as syringes, incontinence pads and colostomy waste cannot be flushed away down the lavatory, neither are they easily burned in domestic boilers or on garden bonfires. Indeed, the Clean Air Act, 1956 may prohibit such activities in certain zones. Disposable syringes are rendered useless by snapping the nozzle and taking care that needles can do no harm; most nursing debris can be wrapped in newspaper or specially provided polythene bags and placed in the dustbin. Liaison in this respect should take place between Environmental Health Inspectors and the primary care team to arrange for the collection of such waste by the dustmen of the local authority's Surveyor's Department.

If the patient requires out-patient treatment or follow up, transport may be required. The Ambulance Service is frequently under pressure and it can be difficult to co-ordinate the timing of the arrival of the ambulance and the readiness of the patient for the journey. For the terminally ill patient such journeys should be only those which are essential and for purposes of treatment which cannot easily be undertaken in the home. It may be easier for the consultant doctor or ward sister to visit the patient's home in the company of the primary care team members. Such action demonstrates an on-going concern for the individual which must surely maintain his confidence in those upon whose skills and knowledge he is totally dependent.

The problem of pain in the dying patient is probably more real when the patient is at home than in the hospital ward. It is well known that pain thresholds in individuals vary and yet doctors and nurses often think that a standard drug régime can apply. Community nurses are frequently very distressed and frustrated at being unable to relieve properly the chronic intractable pain of their patients dying from malignant diseases.

Prescribing drugs is the responsibility of the general practitioner and it should be his earnest endeavour to make this as well planned and effective as possible. The home nursing sister will so arrange her visits that injections can be given at appropriate intervals. If the patient can swallow and is not too nauseated, the relatives should be taught to give correct dosages of oral analgesics and it is helpful if they keep a record for the nurse and family doctor. The nurse, of course, must always record her own drug administration. When the patient lives alone, a system of leaving the correct drug dosages with clear instructions when they are to be taken may need to be devised. It is more common than supposed for such patients to become muddled over the timing and dosage of their medication.

The pioneer work undertaken at St Christopher's Hospice on the control of pain whilst allowing the patient to continue to live his life to the end without constant over-sedation, offers a lesson to us all.

There have been developments in certain parts of the country to provide a twenty-four hour home nursing service. This is a visiting service and has been proved most valuable in the care of the seriously ill and dying. The service requires careful planning, co-operation of family doctors and daytime colleagues, police and the family. Arrangements must be made for the nurse to enter the home at night, but the opportunity to care for patients and the family when they are most vulnerable and alone has been warmly welcomed. This service should be considerably developed.

Nurse managers responsible for community nursing services administer the Marie Curie Memorial Foundation Day and Night Nursing Service on behalf of the Foundation. This makes provision for constant nursing care of patients dying at home from malignant diseases. The Marie Curie nurse becomes part of the team caring for the patient and will frequently 'special' the dying patient in his last days. The provision of comforts and other essentials such as dietary delicacies can be provided by the Marie Curie Memorial Foundation from their welfare grants fund.

Community nurses are well able to advise an appropriate diet for the dying patient. This will usually be easily digested and nourishing, designed in consultation with the family doctor. Should the patient have nausea and frequent vomiting, imagination is required for feeding and carbonated drinks may help. Alcohol may be given with the doctor's permission and egg nogs are nourishing and frequently well tolerated.

Annoxic, disorientated behaviour in the patient can be very distressing to the relatives and may, of course, be a manifestation of the progress of the disease. Medical attention is needed and transfer to hospital care may be indicated if the condition cannot be controlled at home. It is needless to comment that if the patient lives alone alternatives to home care become urgent. At the same time it can be very difficult to arrange, which is another example of the need for inter-team communication and support.

It is appropriate to comment on the development of Community Hospitals. The pilot schemes pioneered in the Oxford Region demonstrate the value of such hospitals for the care of the terminally ill patient. Care continues to be provided by the community-based team within the more easily managed setting of a small hospital unit. Voluntary support from the surrounding community is very real and family and friends can freely participate in the care. It has been noticed that where community ward or hospital facilities are available relatives appear almost eager to relinquish the care of the dying patient, especially as the end approaches, in spite of the fact that underneath it all they might really wish to keep him at home. The decision when to transfer the patient from home to a community hospital, or vice versa, is often more a nursing than a medical decision and the nursing sisters have an important role within the primary care team in this respect. Where good team work exists between doctors and nurses, the opinion of the nurse is valued and accepted.

The value of voluntary workers with the care of the dying has so far been inadequately explored. The commitment has, of necessity, to be on-going. Sporadic help can be given in the form of good neighbour visiting. This is of particular value when the patient is living alone. The potential of involvement within the nursing team of, for example, Red Cross and St John Nursing Volunteers should be tested.

When a patient is in a hospital ward, at least sometime during his stay he will be visited by the hospital chaplain. The community nurse, bound by the nursing ethic to care for patients regardless of race, creed or colour, may often be faced with an overwhelming need by the patient for spiritual comfort. She can offer to mediate between the family and the parish priest. Families are sometimes reluctant to accept his visit either from anxiety lest the patient should discover the true nature of his mortality, or from guilty feelings of past indifference to the church. In many instances, though, much peace of mind and spirit can be gained from pastoral care. Perhaps an extension of the chaplaincy service could be explored.

After the patient has died, the speedy removal of equipment and disposal of unused drugs should be quietly undertaken. Bereavement visiting is an important aspect of the community nurse's work and a close relationship inevitably develops between her and the patient's family. The health visitor may take over this responsibility and will ideally have met the family from time to time during the terminal illness in order to build up an appropriate relationship.

PRESSURES AND PROBLEMS

It must be obvious to the reader that problems in community care of the dying will arise if there is lack of communication or consultation, poor team work and planning, and inadequate resources.

If the nurse requires certain equipment to ensure the right care for her patient, then time lags in the provision and transporting of that equipment to the home will result in inadequate care. If she has too large a case load she cannot give the time she would wish to care of her dying patient. If drugs and medicines are ineffective she cannot help to control pain. If she is not well informed of the patient's condition and prognosis she cannot help to relieve the anxieties of relatives and friends, or properly lead them to accept the reality of losing a loved one with courage.

If the provision of care is of a high standard then to participate in allowing the patient to die in his own home with his family and friends can be one of the most rewarding aspects of community nursing care. The nurse must present a calm and efficient manner and carry out her nursing tasks with all her skill. But never was compassion and loving care more needed, for this with well planned team work can surmount most problems.

And he said:
'You would know the secret of death; But how shall you find it unless you seek it in the heart of life?'

Kahlil Gibran, The Prophet, 1923

REFERENCES

Baly, Monica (1973) *Nursing and Social Change*. London: Heinemann Medical.
Bennett, A. E. (Ed.) (1974) *Community Hospitals: Progress in Development and Evaluation*. Oxford: Oxford Regional Hospital Board.
Care of the Dying. DHSS Reports, No. 5. London: HMSO, 1973.
Cox, Sue (1974) A course in oncology. *Queen's Nursing Journal*, **17**, No. 4, 77.
Desiderata. Old St. Paul's Churchyard, Baltimore, *c.* 1692.
Few, Esme (1969) Survey in Reading on disposal of soiled dressings. *British Hospital Journal and Social Services Review*, **79**, No. 4133, 1247.
Hinton, J. (1974) Talking with people about to die. *British Medical Journal*, **3**, 25.
Marett, Daphne L., Stokes, Mary C. and Simmons, Laurian A. (1973) *Bletchley Night Nursing Pilot Scheme*. Documented by Buckinghamshire County Council Health Department, 14.8.73. (Copies available from Esme Few.)

McNulty, Barbara (1973) The problem of pain in the dying patient. *Queen's Nursing Journal*, **16**, No. 7, 152.

The Care of the Dying Patient and His Family, 1974. Joint Board of Clinical Nursing Studies Course No. 284.

Skeet, Muriel (1970) *Home from Hospital.* London: Dan Mason Nursing Research Committee.

Ward, Audrey W. M. (1974) Telling the patient. *Journal of the Royal College of General Practitioners*, **24**, 465.

7

The Role of the Medical
Social Worker

ANNE KLAR

'THE CENTRAL CHARACTERISTIC of medical social work is its direct concern with the social and emotional problems connected with illness and its medical treatment, and with any consequent adjustments in the lives of patients and their families' (Butrym, 1968). This is particularly necessary when the prognosis of the patient is poor. The social and emotional problems are acutely highlighted to all relatives and staff surrounding the patient, and not least to the patient himself.

A social worker shares with others a real concern for the dying patient and has particular skills which can be used to help both the patient and the family at this time. Since April 1974, the medical social workers in hospitals are on the staff of the local Social Services Departments. There will continue to be discussion on the links between hospitals and local authorities, but the basic training of social workers is the same.

The social workers based in a hospital will be used to working closely with many different professions within the institution. Social workers based outside hospitals are also well accustomed to being part of a network of relationships. Both groups will be concerned with helping their patients through periods of great stress.

THE SOCIAL WORKER IN HOSPITAL

The social worker is not medically trained and has no nursing experience. He or she therefore, does not have the direct physical contact with the patient. This may seem to some to be a deterrent to understanding patients' anxieties. In fact, it is a strength as many patients feel they cannot always talk to a person who is dealing with the often distasteful tasks of bedsores or constant fungating tumours. It is also important that the social worker represents the 'outside' world of a patient—the link with the family and others who have a concept of the patient as a person who has not always been sick. This does not mean that others in the hospital do not have this understanding, but there are often very practical reasons why feelings of this kind are vested in the social worker particularly.

'A fundamental question facing social workers here is, therefore, how to help most effectively when loss is inevitable, or when the possibility of it must be endured for some time? How to help people to deal adequately with their actual or anticipated loss, so that they may become free finally to leave it behind them and to turn to what they still have left with the will and ability to use it fully?

As pain and fear of pain is probably the second most frequent theme in this area of human experience, the social workers have to face a second question; how to help by social work many people who are frightened of suffering?

To pose these questions around loss and fear as social work questions is no denial of the obvious fact that doctors and nurses have heavy responsibilities to help patients and their families in both areas. But the fact is that their major method, that of fighting the illness and seeking a cure, is not available to their lay colleagues; and that many clients can make good use of other methods such as social work, alongside their use of direct medical care' (Snelling, 1962).

Referrals to the medical social worker may come either from the medical or nursing staff, from outside associations, or from the patient. It is essential that the social worker is involved in the team approach and that her role is appreciated by the other members. In some cases it is important that the social worker and doctor see patients together to show their joint appreciation of a patient's anxiety. For instance, a woman who had told the social worker of her fears when facing a mastectomy was able to share this with the surgeon knowing that the social worker was there with her. Equally, a consultant discussing a bad prognosis with relatives may well do this with the social worker who would then share this with them and look at ways of caring for the patient.

The most important part of working with terminally ill patients is sharing with them their feelings. 'Seriously ill patients do consider death as a possible outcome and welcome the chance to talk about their feelings. The fact of sharing this fear . . . is in itself therapeutic and promotes more comfortable communication' (Cramond, 1970).

For example, a young man was referred as he was worried about his financial situation. He had had cardiac surgery which had not been successful and his prognosis was very poor. His first requests were centred around his sickness benefits and detailed queries about allowances for which he was entitled. It soon became clear that although he was talking about his present situation he was beginning to think about his family's future. He was becoming aware of his own deterioration and with it came a sense of worthlessness at being unable to fulfil his own expectations of himself. By gradually helping the patient to look at the reality of his financial situation, seeking ways through funds to meet outstanding bills, the social worker was able to help him feel that he was still able to retain his role as head of the family. At the same time the social worker came to know his wife and share with her the fears of the future. Finally, very near the end of the patient's life there was a joint interview in which the patient and his wife openly acknowledged the fears and anxieties of them both, with the knowledge of the on-going support of the social worker.

Some patients cannot discuss their feelings and problems so easily. They ask for help in different ways. A physical illness may necessitate looking at and working on the whole life of the patient. A middle-aged woman was knocked down and brought to the casualty department. She had no injuries from the accident, but was found to have a large fungating carcinoma of the breast. She was referred to the social worker as she had refused admission 'for social reasons'.

Away from the pressures of the casualty department she was able to reveal gradually her real anxiety of leaving her husband alone because of his alcoholic problem. In her anxiety at 'protecting' him she had not felt able to consider her own health. She was also so frightened of her condition that her husband's problems provided a way for her to avoid making a decision about treatment. The social worker having gained the confidence of the patient and assessed the various needs, was able to move ahead and, with the assistance of a family doctor, help that patient into hospital; also, she could start to help the husband to agree to treatment and thus share and appreciate his wife's anxiety.

These examples show the ways in which a social worker assesses and works with the problems of terminal illness within the hospital setting. Moving at the pace that a patient can accept and being aware of the changing needs is of fundamental importance.

The social worker will often be involved with very practical ways of helping the patient. A thorough knowledge of the Social Service is essential; for instance the extra payments that can be made from Supplementary Benefits Commission in terms of grants for special diets or extra heating. In certain circumstances there can be weekly grants from the National Society for Cancer Relief to help with extra food, or to meet a special need like a separate bed for the patient. The Welfare Department of the Marie Curie Memorial Foundation will help with special grants for many domiciliary needs of patients with malignant diseases. If these sources of help are used imaginatively it can be of inestimable help to patients and their families. However, alongside the provision of services must be the ability to accept them.

A patient or relative may ask a social worker about problems which are clearly outside her professional skill; for instance facts about nursing procedures or 'medical' information. This is sometimes because the patient has been unable to ask the appropriate person, or maybe was afraid to do so. To a sick person the experience and competence of staff can be a frightening experience. A social worker will need to be able to pick up these points and help the patient make the request directly or act as an 'interpreter' for him.

This is particularly the case when discussing terminal care with relatives. Often it may seem that they are talking 'remotely' about the patient's death, funeral arrangements, etc. Often this is a defensive way of dealing with the real emotional problems they know they will be facing and the support they will need to give the other members of the family. For example, the husband of a young woman with three children talked at length about giving up his job, changing his house and moving the children's schools. The social worker considered all these ideas with him, and basically acknowledged his need to reflect on his changing life pattern. In fact none of these drastic things needed to happen; but his mourning, started before his wife's death, was a necessary part of his preparation.

There are patients who cannot return home in their terminal stage. This may be because of the nature of the nursing care needed, or they have no home to go to. Sometimes it is because relatives cannot stand the physical and emotional strain involved. Decisions about appropriate after-care are usually the result of joint discussion between medical, nursing and social work staff. Experience of joint interviews in this way has been very positive. The doctor shares his concern about the patient's future and explains the medical needs and the social worker follows this by a time of reflection on this information and its meaning to the family.

Sometimes this delicate work is left to the family doctor who knows the family and it is therefore important to have good liaison with the social work staff in hosptal.

Provisions for continuing in-patient care vary greatly throughout the country. There are, unfortunately, a limited number of specialised homes such as those of the Marie Curie Memorial Foundation and St Christopher's Hospice. Wherever possible it is helpful for relatives to go and see the home before the patient is admitted there. This gives a chance for certain fantasies of somebody 'being put away' to be explored and often makes admission much easier. This also means that a relative can tell the patient of this visit and so it becomes a joint decision. The fears of rejection by the hospital are very real at this time and the ways in which various members of the hospital staff can help with this always need consideration.

Unfortunately, it is not always possible to make the ideal placement, either because of lack of facilities or an acute shortage of beds. Too often the social worker has to make *ad hoc* arrangements at the last minute. This often means additional pressure on domiciliary services and severe anxiety on the patient and relative. The provision of more specialised facilities could prevent ill prepared patients feeling thrust away by the parent hospital at their time of greatest need. It might also do much to prevent some of the mental ill health which often follows in the form of depression when relatives have not had a chance to prepare for death, or feel guilty at not having cared sufficiently for the patient.

Thus, a social worker in hospital works with the medical and nursing staff to help patients and families at a crisis point in their lives. She uses her skills to help people come to terms with their situation and to manipulate their environment, as far as possible, and to enable them to accept and use the many different forms of help available.

THE SOCIAL WORKER OUTSIDE HOSPITAL

The social worker based outside hospital works in the same way but may approach the problem differently. To her, illness is one facet of a person's life, whereas her colleague in the hospital will see this as the factor which introduced her to the patient. Similarly, the social worker may not have the day to day medical knowledge and may require more interpretation of this from medical and nursing staff.

A social worker will bring knowledge of family and personal dynamics and how people deal with stress. There may have been many crises within the family and the point of the social worker's intervention hitherto could have been the mental illness of one member, problems about the children, or care of an elderly relative. This kind of knowledge is a very valuable asset in the total care of the patient and the family at a time when they are experiencing another form of stress.

'It can be very hard to carry on with life when someone close is approaching the end of theirs. One feels guilty. It is so poignant, and thus so difficult to attend to things like children's birthdays, starting a new school or a new job, keeping wedding anniversaries or the deeply private anniversaries of significant times of married life. The social worker helps the family to hold to a balance between the "going on living" events of family life, and the preparation for losing the person who is dying' (Daniel, 1972).

The changing sociological pattern of the country is such that it is possible that families are scattered and do not have the support of nearby relatives. Also with the increased life expectancy, it is not so common for a young person to have experienced death within the family. This can also be the case with people living in an urban community away from the close-knit village situation. Death is then not only a deep emotional experience, but also a new one for many.

It is these aspects of life and death which a social worker will be sharing with the patient wherever he or she may be. The role of the social worker with the terminally ill is a vital one, together with the other caring professions. She will use her skills to enable a patient to benefit to the maximum from medical care and to retain until the last a quality of life.

REFERENCES

Butrym, Zophia (1968) *Social Work in Medical Care.* London: Routledge & Kegan Paul.
Cramond, W. A. (1970) Psychotherapy of the dying patient. *British Medical Journal,* 3, 389.
Daniel, M. P. (1972) In *Care of the Dying.* DHSS Reports, No. 5. London: HMSO, 1973.
Snelling, Jean (1962) Social work within medical care. *The Almoner* (June).

8

Personal Observations

GERALD WHITE MILTON

THIS CHAPTER[1] is concerned primarily with the care of a dying adult who would normally expect many more years of life. It is not concerned with the death of infants, sudden accidental death or the anti-mortem care of the senile.

Knowledge of an approaching death affects a group of people. At the centre of the group is the patient; the first circle about him is made up of his nearest relatives; the second circle surrounding the patient are those in professional contact with him, doctors, lawyers, priests, etc., the third circle includes home nursing services and a large variety of para-medical personnel; somewhat more to the periphery forming a fourth circle about the patient are his workmates, his employer or employees and beyond this again is the indifferent or curious general public.

The care of the patient falls naturally under two headings:

1. The care of organic illness
2. The emotional and psychological care of the patient and his family.

I will not discuss the care of organic disease here. The emotional care of the patient and his family is dealt with by first considering the emotions in the mind of a patient who develops fatal illness and then considering the ways and means of helping him and his family.

THOUGHTS IN THE MIND OF A PATIENT SUFFERING FROM A FATAL ILLNESS

The thoughts in the mind of a patient with incurable disease usually pass through different stages and at each stage the patient and his relatives have to adjust to changing circumstances by a

[1]Milton, 1972, 1973a and 1973b.

variety of techniques. The amount of suffering by the group may be increased by thoughtless or clumsy management.

Stage 1
The attitude of a person to the knowledge of a potentially fatal illness will initially be influenced by the way the disease presents. From the patient's point of view fatal illness may present in one of two ways.

First, a perfectly healthy man goes to a doctor thinking he has a trivial complaint, and a small operation or a bottle of medicine is all that is required to put him right. When in the doctor's consulting room the doctor discovers signs or symptoms which suggests a disease which could be fatal, for example, cancer, if the doctor exclaims his diagnosis, 'You've got a growth in there', the patient in his own mind passes from health to an unexpected death sentence in moments. 'Instant cancer'. Each of us requires a minimal time to adjust our thoughts to personal disasters.

The second method of presentation of fatal illness is for the patient to become aware of persistent and slowly worsening symptoms. The patient suspects that he has a serious illness by the time he visits his doctor. When a fatal disease presents in this way the time required for mental acclimatisation to personal misfortune has been provided by the slow progress of the disease.

In Stage 1 the patient's emotional feelings are those of apprehension about the diagnosis. The ease with which he adjusts to the diagnosis of a dangerous and possibly fatal illness depends on his personality and the manner of presentation of the disease.

Stage 2
When the diagnosis is established one of the adjustments the patient must make is to recognise the fact that he has a malignancy or a potentially fatal illness. Most of us imagine that unpleasant diseases, like malignancy, affect others but not ourselves. This protective denial is extensively used to deal with problems. A person who smokes heavily secretly thinks that he will not get a cancer but others might. A reckless driver really does not anticipate getting killed but other fast drivers might. So the patient with incurable illness has to become reconciled to the fact that 'This time it's *me*'. The difficulty of adjustment to this situation is displayed by the patient who says, 'I can't believe this is happen-

ing to me, it feels like a bad dream.' The next feeling, as the horrible truth sinks in, is best described by the patient's question— 'Why me? What have I done to deserve this? I have never harmed anyone.' The patient now has only a short step to sink into a morass of self-pity. At the same time as this happens he develops a resentment against his fate which may be centred on his healthy spouse, 'You don't know what I have got to go through'; 'You don't care what happens to me.'

As these feelings develop the patient becomes increasingly cantankerous and irritable. The irritability, as a rule, is not displayed to those professionally taking care of him. I presume this is so because the doctor is the last thread of hope the patient possesses. The irritability seems to be greatest towards his nearest family, where the feeling may become so marked as to become jealousy. When this happens the spouse through no fault of her own cannot do anything right. As the emotional adjustment proceeds through these stages and as the inevitability of death sinks into the patient he tends to become alone and isolated from people around him.

One factor which increases the patient's irritability may be the increasing suspicion that his wife and his doctor are deceiving him.

Stage 3
Another prominent emotion as the disease advances is fear. The patient is frightened of several things, of being dead; of the process of dying and of pain; suffering and lack of dignity; and, naturally, he has a great feeling of sadness of leaving loved ones and happy associations. Fear of being dead is a subject so universal that nearly all religious beliefs endeavour to reassure believers that there is a second life. Fear of the process of dying is often increased by the fact that in modern Western society the only personal association with death for most people will have been the demise of an elderly senile relative. The slow process of disintegration and the gradual conversion of a human being into a 'thing' is alarming to anyone who believes he is on the same road. The fear of uncontrollable pain is both common and understandable. The doctor can promise his patient that modern methods of pain relief can eliminate even the most severe pains.

If a surgical operation is advised for treatment the patient will often be frightened at the prospect but ashamed to acknowledge it.

So he will cover up his dread of the treatment by such remarks as, 'Of course, I'm not worried for myself doctor. I have had a good life, but I really am worried about the wife and children'. The more strenuously the patient stresses his worries for his family to the doctor the more he displays fear for himself. Apprehension for his next of kin is a common feeling of the fatally ill, especially if the patient and his family are young; but the patient will usually express these fears to his wife and not so much to his doctor.

Stage 4
As the last stage of this 'strange eventful history' is reached, the main dread of the patient is being cut off from life. This shows itself in the patient's behaviour, which often seems to recede into childishness, and dependence on objects and people around him. It may be highly desirable for the patient to be in hospital so that he can be given care and attention throughout the day and night. As the ambulance draws up outside his home he feels that he will be carried out never to see his life's pleasures again. So he will not leave. Alternatively the patient may develop a child-like dependence on doctors and nurses and be most reluctant to leave 'you wonderful people'. The young doctor may feel flattered when his patient says repeatedly that the staff in the hospital are wonderful; the resident medical officer (intern) is wonderful and that the surgeon is so marvellously clever that he must be the greatest man in his field, etc. Any doctor or nurse would be hardly human if they were not gratified with such glowing praise. Most patients are genuinely grateful to all members of the team for their efforts on his behalf. But, beware, if the effusion of praise and gratitude is excessive because such patients are often really bolstering their own apprehensions. The cleverer the medical team, the greater the chance of cure.

One emotion, always on the sidelines and which may come to dominate the patient, is depression which is hardly surprising under the circumstances.

The Spouse's Feelings
As the illness of the husband develops his wife passes through several stages of apprehension. First, she dimly realises that he is not well, but reassures herself that he has been overworking. As his condition deteriorates she begins to fear the worst, so she wants to

visit the doctor with him. 'One can always face up to things if one accepts them openly, without deception.' But no sooner has the doctor told her the truth she fears than she seeks to protect her husband. 'We must never tell him, he couldn't stand it.' The second stage begins when she has to lead a double life telling the truth to everybody (relatives, workmates, etc.) except the person most concerned (her husband). Their relationship, therefore, develops into a game, each trying to manoeuvre the other into believing something false while both know the truth. The wife is therefore torn two ways, and it is hardly surprising that the strain begins to take effect.

The patient's wife has the added burden of grief, and may find the prospect of life alone without her husband too horrible to contemplate.

If the patient has an open wound or colostomy requiring attention, the untrained members of the family may be so revolted by the appearance that they cannot force themselves to attend to it. This is not purely weakness of character or lack of feeling, it is simply an extension of the fact that some people faint at the sight of blood and others do not.

The husband's episodes of irritability are most distressing because the wife feels guilty if she relaxes her attention for a moment. She may have real anxiety for herself, 'I really don't know what I will do after he is gone. I haven't enough money to live on. I don't know what will happen to me.' So as the illness progresses his wife suffers physical fatigue and emotional strain. If the game of denial of the facts of death is played by the patient, his wife and doctor to its limit, then the effects of bereavement tend to be more severe when it is impossible to ignore the truth any longer. (Maddison, 1968).

Failure of communication between different members of the team caring for a dying patient may influence the distress of the bereaved (Maddison, 1968). Close relatives of the dead patient may feel anger and resentment against the medical personnel if communication has been inadequate.

There are, of course, some spouses who relish the idea of being a widow and their good health and cheerfulness never falter as the patient slowly melts into his grave. Needless to say the husband in this situation is more likely than ever to show self-pity and resentment.

The Patient's Children

The suffering patient is torn two ways about his children. He may want them to remember him in his prime and not as they will see him on his decline to death. Alternatively his wish to see his children, talk to them and retain a feeling that his own life continues in them may be so overpowering that he wants them near him as much as possible.

The patient's wife is also in a dilemma. She fears that the sight of sickness may permanently upset the children but she appreciates her husband's wish that they should be near. The children themselves seem to react in one of two ways. If the truth has always been avoided they are mystified, but of course, sense tragedy. If they are told the truth and face it they are surprisingly good at handling the situation, even when very young.

I believe it is a mistake to send the children away or to try to deceive them. It is also, I believe, a mistake to tell them the truth but at the same time say they must on no account talk about it to their father. I have a friend who was given this advice when his father was dying of cancer. He said many times since his father's death he wished he had been allowed to talk freely in a realistic way for there were so many things he wanted to say that he was not allowed to mention.

Children are much more resilient than their parents sometimes give them credit for. They can accept the truth far better than a game of fantasy which they know is false.

MANAGEMENT

If the foregoing is an accurate picture of the feelings of a family when a fatal illness affects one of its members; how should the medical team behave towards the family to help them in their distress? This is just as important a part of medicine as examining a chest or abdomen or prescribing an antibiotic.

The team who manage a dying patient consists of the following:

1. A consultant physician, surgeon, or radiotherapist, etc.
2. A local family doctor
3. Nursing staff of a hospital ward or out-patient department
4. Social worker of a hospital or clinic
5. A minister of religion

6. The patient's family
7. His colleagues or superiors at work

It is important to make this a team and not seven individuals or groups pulling different ways. The leader of the team may change from time to time but the first six members listed here should communicate with each other and with the patient freely and effectively enough for them to understand and to trust one another.

The management of the dying should start at the first interview between doctor (family doctor or consultant) and patient. If a family doctor suspects that his patient has a potentially fatal disease he should insist that husband and wife attend the consultant together. If this has not been done and the consultant suspects a potentially fatal illness he should arrange a second interview with the patient and his wife together. The reason for this is that there must be a frank and honest relationship between the team members and the patient. It is hard enough at any time to establish effective communication and almost impossible to do so if the first encounters of the members of the group make them suspicious that one or other is holding back unpleasant information.

If the consultant senses that the patient has no idea that he could have any form of fatal illness then the patient must have time to become mentally adjusted to his diagnosis. This is simply done by deferring a detailed discussion about the treatment until all investigations are complete; the patient having the ultimate diagnosis suggested by some remark such as, 'This could be more serious than it seems, but I must get some tests done first before we talk it over in detail.'

A truthful bond between surgeon, patient, his wife and the family doctor therefore, starts at their first or second encounter, long before the possibility of dying is seriously considered; that is at a stage when the patient is apprehensive about the diagnosis.

As the patient moves into the next stage when the diagnosis is established, but cure is still a reasonable anticipation, some relatives plead that the patient should not be told he has cancer. This is well-meant but wrong. My answer to this remark is something as follows: 'I understand that you want to protect your husband (father) from bad news about himself, but I have had more experience in dealing with this problem than you and although you know your husband (father) so well, I assure you that if you try to deceive him you will only make his suffering worse. We will see him together and we can talk over his problem frankly as adults.' At the interview every effort is made to stress the positive and hopeful aspects of the patient's condition, but deliberate lying is avoided. I do not know of any family who regretted this course of action after it had been carried out.

In Stage 2 although the diagnosis was frankly discussed with the patient at an earlier interview the patient may protect himself with a total denial of his condition. If this happens it is neither necessary nor desirable to break down the protective barrier. But if the patient starts to look for truth he must be given it in a humane form. The patient's other feelings in Stage 2, 'Why me?', suspicion, jealousy and irritability are again helped by frank honesty and even drawing his attention to his wife's suffering, 'You and your wife are having a worrying time, try to think of her a bit if you can, you can help her quite a lot.' In this way turn the subject from the patient to the distressed relatives and make the dying patient feel something for his immediate family. This cannot always be done but one has to try to redirect the egocentricity of the patient outward from himself. The patient should never have grounds for feeling that he has been deceived. A remark like, 'You wouldn't tell me even if I had cancer, would you?' should never need to be made against the doctor.

Beware of pity. The mournful face, the gloomy remark, 'I am *so* sorry for you', do the patient no good and merely drive him to self-pity. In other words, there is a balance of commonsense; kindness is not achieved by avoiding unpleasant subjects, or expressing sympathy.

The general fear of the patient may be partly alleviated by a good team. Fear of being dead is not a medical problem. Fear of dying is partly alleviated by telling the patient that you will never desert him, that any time he wants to ask questions you will try to answer them. The fear of pain and the lack of dignity have been dealt with. The patient's dread of the effects of treatment can be helped partly by the doctor responsible for treatment, for example, the consultant and partly by the presence of the patient's wife at the interview when it is discussed. The bond of a successful marriage is of the greatest help at this time. The wife can reassure the husband that the operation will not affect her feelings for him,

D

that she will be near him, etc. It is hard to explain how this can help a patient, but it does. At other times in this interview the patient may support his wife with encouraging words. The combined interview avoids the patient feeling alone.

The fear of loss of personal dignity is often increased because the patient has been in hospital before and seen how a terminal patient was ignored by the staff. A ward sister stands at the foot of the dying man's bed and says to a junior nurse, 'This patient is to be turned every two hours, nurse' and moves on. The consultant may say to the resident (but loud enough for the patient and those near him to hear), 'Nothing to be done here Dr X', and again moves on without a backward glance. If a patient is nearing the end of his life it is as important as ever to take seriously any of his complaints. For example, if a terminal cancer patient complains of backache, the site should be examined by the consultant, who should also listen carefully to the patient's history. The conduct of all of us in hospital wards is always observed by other patients, and although one does not play to the gallery one should not ignore those patients for whom cure is no longer possible.

The management of depression is difficult because its cause cannot be remedied. The Melanoma Clinic at Sydney Hospital has a psychiatrist permanently attached to it and his help with the depressed is invaluable. I should also point out here that in a cancer clinic the junior staff can be helped by group discussions in the presence of a psychiatrist.

The stresses and strains on the wife of a dying man have been mentioned earlier in this chapter. One point remains, when the patient is at home the wife is on duty twenty-four hours a day. She sleeps in the same room as the sick man and day after day is worried about the patient, her children, and herself. She may also feel guilty if she fails (or thinks she has failed) in any of her duties to her dying husband. Any person subjected to this strain for more than a few weeks is bound to come near to breakdown. Hence, the doctor must see that the wife is relieved to allow her at least a few hours each week away from the sick bed. It is useless to try to stimulate the spouse into greater effort, she is already driven by her own feelings, if she is an average person. Of course, if the wife is indifferent to her husband's distress, threats will not do any good. Thus, in all cases other family members must be used to help out.

The most peripheral rings around the dying patient are made up of his company and workmates, and of the indifferent or curious general public. The public is entertained by death in two forms, the spectacular and the horrible. A death occurring quietly in bed from natural causes has little impact on the 'man in the street'. Large business concerns are often believed to be vast and heartless machines, as indeed they probably are to the inefficient employee. However, when the final days of a man's life are at hand it has been my experience that even the larger companies will do all that is reasonable to help the patient and his family. It is well worthwhile including some members of the patient's business firm from time to time in the team which cares for him and his family.

The last thing to consider is the doctor's point of view. The management of terminal disease is often badly handled by the medical profession for several reasons. Death underlines the failure of medicine. A doctor usually does not associate himself with his patient's illness because it is easy for him to believe that he will never have the patient's disease. But the doctor cannot deny that he will die. Death is unavoidable, so all who come in contact with the fatally ill know that it is only a matter of time before they will follow the patient to the grave. This fact makes it more difficult to stand detached from the dying. It is more comfortable for the doctor and the team to avoid the idea that they are also mortal and as this cannot be done with the process of dying, it may be accomplished by avoiding dying patients. This may make the doctor or his staff more comfortable for a while, but it would not be in the interests of either his patient or of medicine as a whole.

REFERENCES

Milton, G. W. (1972) The care of the dying. *Medical Journal of Australia*, **2**, 177.
Milton, G. W. (1973a) Self willed death or the bone pointing syndrome. *Lancet*, **i**, 1435.
Milton, G. W. (1973b) Thoughts in the mind of a person with cancer. *British Medical Journal*, **4**, 5886.
Maddison, D. (1968) The relevance of conjugal bereavement for preventative psychiatry. *British Journal of Medical Psychology*, **41**, 223.

9

Teaching About Death and Dying:
An Interdisciplinary Approach
MICHAEL A. SIMPSON

IN SEVERAL WAYS, the dying represent one of the most neglected minority groups in modern medicine. Generally, any patients who are perceived by the medical and nursing staff as unattractive and hard to help, as threatening to their personal preconceptions or prejudices, or who arouse uncomfortable feelings in the health professional, are likely to be neglected, crudely or subtly. Such patients include the old, the psychiatrically ill and mentally subnormal, the sexually and socially deviant, the homeless and the dying. Philosophically, one of the factors delineating man as a human being has been his capacity to recognise the inevitability of death. But although this fact may be intellectually acknowledged, this is usually with the working assumption that death is something that happens to other people. It is much more difficult to recognise and come to terms with our own mortality.

ATTITUDES TO DEATH AND THE NEED FOR TEACHING

The management of dying patients can arouse intense emotional turmoil in medical and nursing staff, which can result in various forms of direct and indirect avoidance of the patient. This not only generates considerable personal anxiety, but it leads to difficulty in accurately recognising the patient's psychological, social, spiritual and even physical needs, and impaired patient care. Feifel and his colleagues (1967) have reported, although further substantiation of their findings is needed, that although a group of physicians they tested appeared to think rather less about death than did two control groups of patients and of non-professionals, they appeared to be more afraid of death than either of the control groups. Feifel's hypothesis was that a major factor influencing some physicians to enter medicine was the need to master their own above-average fears of death.

Saul and Kass (1969) studied junior medical students in Boston, and asked them to rank fifteen specific situations they were expected to encounter in their first year, by the amount of anxiety they expected to feel in the situation. The two most anxiety-provoking and feared situations were related to death, discussing a fatal illness with a patient and telling a relative that a patient had died.

Several major factors influence attitudes to death among members of the health professions. One is the almost total lack of suitable teaching, or even opportunities to discuss the subject, until very recently. Dying is after all an even more universal experience than sex, and although problems related to one or both of these vital areas are extremely common, medical students have had to graduate knowing no more about either subject than they knew when they arrived at medical school, gleaned from their significantly limited personal experiences.

Another major factor influencing professional attitudes to death is the increasingly limited relevant experience they seem to have had prior to their training. Knutson in 1968 studied a group of health professionals, and found that only 30 per cent had experienced a death in the family, and just 15 per cent had witnessed a death before starting professional training.

The author (1973a; 1973b) studied a group of student nurses in London and found that 8 per cent had not seen a dead body, and 35 per cent had never witnessed a death, even during their training. Those that had, mainly noticed in passing the unexpected (and therefore not tidied away) death of an old stranger, in hospital. Only 12 per cent had experienced the death of a member of the family and only 8 per cent had been present at a death. In response to a question on attitudes to funerals, over 20 per cent additionally volunteered that they had never seen one. Thirty-five per cent had the opportunity to talk about death at home, and while most made use of every opportunity for informal discussions about it, only 11 per cent had had any formal chance to do so while at school, and only 22 per cent found the chance during their nursing training.

Probably in no other clinical area do health professionals' attitudes and personal experiences have such an influence on patient care. Yet they are seldom offered the opportunity to discuss and understand their personal beliefs and responses, or to receive help in managing difficult cases in this area. I know of cases in which nursing staff found dying patients' expressions of distress intolerable, and responded to the patients' urgent attempts to talk about their fears of dying by requesting a marked increase in the dosage of analgesics (although the patient was suffering no major physical pain), treating tears with opiates until the patient was once more suitably quiescent and silent. Let us not give the patient morphine for our own pain.

There are several ways in which we seem to apply double standards. For example, although as many as 80 per cent of doctors in some surveys say that patients should not be told that they have cancer; some 60 per cent say that they would of course want to be told if they themselves had cancer. Among the nurses I studied (Simpson, 1973a; 1973b), the position was subtly different. Seventy-six per cent said they would want to be told that they were dying, while 98 per cent said they believed that patients should be told they are dying, if they wish to know. But 70 per cent would personally avoid telling a patient he had any unfavourable diagnosis. The nurses, therefore, had an advantage doctors lacked, in that they could believe in telling a patient his prognosis without feeling obliged to do so themselves. Doctors, on the other hand, tend to see themselves as in charge of the information and its distribution. We may talk about the patient's diagnosis, but we treat the diagnosis as if it belonged to us.

THE INTERDISCIPLINARY APPROACH

It is beginning to be recognised that good patient care needs efficient co-ordination between the different members of the health care team. With regard to the care of the dying patient, this may mean principally the doctor, the nurse, the social worker and the chaplain, but may also involve nursing assistants, ward receptionists, aides, technicians, students, porters and maids. In the out-patient and home care of the patient, others may be involved including out-patient staff; district nurses; in North America, nurse practitioners; and voluntary agencies. Dying children involve further personnel, such as teachers and counsellors, play therapists, and psychologists. It is not merely paying lip-service to the currently fashionable team concept, to describe the involvement of such a variety of persons, for any or all of them can have an important part to play in terminal care. In one major London teaching hospital I know, for example, a talented and warmly humane ward receptionist spends more time with the dying, and gives them more comfort, than any member of the medical or social work staff.

We should not forget, either, that in the proper management of any disease, and particularly acutely with terminal illness, the patient's family and friends may in a very real sense be appropriate members of the team.

INTERDISCIPLINARY TEACHING

Wherever possible, I try to ensure that all the teaching sessions I take part in on this subject, are organised on an interdisciplinary basis. At the undergraduate level, this may involve medical, nursing and social work students and, where possible, sociology, psychology and divinity students. At the postgraduate level any of the various personnel mentioned above may with profit be involved. Especially in a seminar or small group setting, considerable student support and enthusiasm can be generated and all participants can learn from each other. I believe it is appropriate in many instances to train together students from different disciplines who are going to work together in the future. They can be enabled to gain an increased understanding of the differing attitudes, experiences, problems and role-perceptions of their colleagues, which can help them to have more realistic mutual expectations, and improve the chances of effective co-operation as an integrated team after graduation.

Interest in interdisciplinary teaching in general is increasing, and my experience suggests that this is a particularly suitable area for the development of such programmes. Interdisciplinary teaching is most successful when it is problem-based rather than subject-based, when it incorporates small group problem-solving, dealing with clinical and biomedical problems in whose management the different disciplines have different approaches and expertise. It is least successful when based on traditional subject boundaries such as 'anatomy', where the disciplines may vary in the amount of the subject they need to use, the depth required to understand it, and in the substance of the subject itself. Also, such interdisciplinary programmes should probably not be organised very early in the curriculum, with students newly entered upon their training. Such teaching is in fact only nominally or pseudo-interdisciplinary when the participants have not yet begun to differentiate or learn varying role-models. The integration of students at such an early stage when there is still more variation in life experiences *among* medical students, for example, than *between* medical students and nurses, is simply not worth the often heroic administrative contortions that may be required in many modern institutions just to arrange for both groups to get to the same place at the same time.

DEATH AND DYING: THE STATE OF THE ART

It has become a cliché to state that we live in a death-denying society. Largely, this is still true; but we appear to be entering a transitional phase, and recent years have seen a dramatic interest in all aspects of death. Death has yet to reach the state of tawdry public ubiquity that sex has suffered, but a very similar trend is discernible. Among the valuable publications which have undoubtedly advanced our understanding of the subject, we have seen the publication of an increasing number of repetitious and duplicative books and articles, and the beginnings of frankly exploitative works. While valuable and artistically significant films have been produced and more are needed, the film industry at large is beginning to produce movies that flirt with death as tastelessly as their sexploitation equivalents.

The expansion of general interest in the subject has been impressive. Ten years ago, a competent bibliographer listed some 400 published items for the book *Death and Identity* (Fulton, 1965). The most recently published bibliography (Fulton, 1973) lists over 2,600 items.

Schoenberg and Carr in 1972 reported the results of an earlier survey of sixty-eight American medical schools, conducted by the Foundation of Thanatology. Almost half of those replying reported that the requirements for the diagnosis of death were not formally included in their curriculum. Over one third stated that the doctor's responsibility for the care of the dying patient's family and of the bereaved, was not included. Relatively few reported themselves as being satisfied with their teaching efforts in this respect, yet only one third indicated plans for curricular changes to improve the situation. Examination questions on the subject were effectively unknown.

Liston in 1973 made a survey of education on death and dying in American medical schools, and I have recently completed a survey of British medical schools (Simpson, 1975). Liston identified forty-one schools with formal or structured programmes for the instruction of medical students in the psychological care and understanding of patients with fatal illnesses. Nearly 90 per cent of the programmes had been in existence for more than five years. Sixty-four per cent were required; of those which were elective, the proportion of eligible students who chose to take them varied from 1–50 per cent, averaging 15 per cent. Most of them (73 per cent) were for medical students exclusively, but the remainder were integrated with a wide variety of other disciplines. About a quarter were exclusively lectures, over half consisted primarily of seminars; the remainder combined both techniques. Seventy per cent featured at least one interview with a dying patient, and most allowed the students the opportunity of interviewing patients. Students' evaluations of such courses were reported to be positive; 57 per cent rating them as highly valuable, 27 per cent as of moderate value and 9 per cent as of some value.

In Britain, I received replies from twenty-five of the twenty-nine schools, an 84 per cent response. Of those schools responding, 68 per cent offered formal teaching on death, mostly (36 per cent) using a combination of lectures, seminars and bedside teaching; 20 per cent relied on one or two lectures. Another 20 per cent, incorporated visits to units specialising in terminal care, although only one formally provided opportunities to interview and get to know dying patients. Forty-four per cent specified that their teaching was exclusively for medical students, and only two schools had any interdisciplinary teaching except informally and extra-curricular, in debates and meetings arranged by medical student societies, and the London Medical Group and similar groups in Glasgow and Newcastle. When offered an index of satisfaction with the current state of teaching, a great majority of schools indicated that they were 'mildly satisfied', with true British understatement. Twenty-four per cent of schools planned some extension of teaching in this area. In 28 per cent of schools, the teaching was both regular and required; 20 per cent indicated that it had, at some point, featured in final examinations. The subjects most frequently taught were the legal and certification aspects, covered in all but one of the schools which dealt with death. The role of other health care workers featured considerably less often (only 44 per cent of courses); and the care of the bereaved was somewhat less frequently taught (56 per cent).

EXPERIENCES OF DEATH

In the absence of formal teaching, students are greatly influenced by their encounters with death in medical school, and I have explored this in small group discussions with students in several countries. There is a succession of memorable experiences, usually starting with dissection. It is usually less upsetting than the student anticipated, as the cadaver is less than insistently human, due to preservatives and post-mortem changes. As one student cited by Barton (1972) said, 'That first cut through the skin is really bad; but when you get down there and it begins to look like the anatomy book, and it doesn't look like a human being anymore, it's not so bad'. Dissection of some parts of the body which are harder to reify and dehumanise, the hands, eyes, and genitalia, may remain upsetting. The next significant experience is the autopsy, where the more vivid colouring and smells of the body, its freshness and the relative immediacy of death, produces increased anxiety. Later, the student experiences the autopsy of a patient he has known while alive, which may renew the anxiety. The tendency is to move towards an increasingly impersonal and technical view of the whole death situation. As a manoeuvre of defence this may be successful in managing the intense feelings aroused by threatening situations, though it may impair patient care in some instances. Rough and nervous jokes are also seen as a common defensive technique, such as the sequence of 'How do you break the news to a patient?' jokes; for example, 'Put it this way, Mr. Johnson—don't buy any long-playing records'.

Later, usually in the internship, come the first occasions when the young doctor is called to the bedside to certify death. Commonly, he may return to his bed in the small hours of the morning, apprehensively awaiting the call that will tell him that the patient he has just certified has sat up in the mortuary. The junior doctor may also be surprised at the extent of his hostility towards patients when over-tired.

TEACHING ABOUT DEATH AND DYING

Methods and Examples

So far, the literature provides little help, advice or guidance for those wishing to start a teaching programme on this subject. The bibliography on page 104 lists what appears to be the entire literature on the subject, apart from those articles cited in this chapter. Barton (1972) has written about the need for such teaching in medical school, based on some small group discussions he had held with medical students as part of a second year psychiatry course. Later he and his colleagues (1972) described an elective course on Psychosocial Aspects of Life-Threatening Illness, for third and fourth year students; a comprehensive sequence of one hour seminars once a week for a sixteen week semester. Olin (1972) published some suggestions for a model programme, but this was not based on personal experience, and was purely speculative. Liston (1974) has described a course on Psychiatric Aspects of Life-Threatening Illness, for students during their clinical clerkship in psychiatry, and consisting of four or five seminars and patient interviews. Preston (1973) described courses in Ageing, Retirement and Mortality for the general public.

As an example of a larger and more ambitious programme, we can consider the interdisciplinary course I have run at McMaster University in Canada. The following were among the objectives of the programme, drawn up after discussion with prospective participants. The participants should:

Become familiar with the available evidence and range of opinions, on death, dying, and bereavement;

Develop the capacity to relate the subjects covered, to their personal feelings about these emotionally charged subjects; become more aware of the nature and range of their feelings; consider their personal mortality and fears of death and how their feelings influence their behaviour towards patients;

Improve their facility for expressing such feelings and fears, and become more aware of such feelings in others, including other members of the health care team; to consider how they could handle strong differences of opinion with other members of the team.

Begin to develop communication skills with respect to talking with dying patients, and competency in dealing with the practical problems of dying and bereavement, in their own most appropriate clinical setting.

Explore some aspects of the multidisciplinary approach to learning and patient care; develop a clearer concept of their role in their own discipline, and of the roles, needs, and perceptions of members of other professions and disciplines;

Develop a critical awareness of current practices in the care of the dying, the bereaved, and the dead.

The programme combined large and small group experiences. Once a week from March through May, a sequence of large group sessions lasting 60–90 minutes presented a variety of information and experiences around a given theme. Themes ranged from 'Personal Mortality, The Health Care Team and the Care of the Dying', 'Children and Death', 'Ageing and the Approach of Death', 'Moral, Ethnical and Legal Aspects of Death', Comparative Religions and Funeral Practices', to 'Bereavement'. A variety of techniques were used. In one session for example, a mixed-media presentation prepared with the participation of some of the class, combined poetry, music, film, prose and dramatic excerpts, in illustrating some of the many approaches to the different facets of death.

In another session, following a presentation of the facts of current morbidity statistics—who dies, when, and where, and the cause—each student opened an envelope given to him earlier, and found a death certificate in his name. They were asked to fill it in as they expected their own certificate would in time be completed. Two studies of this technique have been made (Sabatini and Kastenbaum, 1973; Simpson, 1974) and it not only personifies the fact of personal mortality dramatically, but reveals the extent of denial of the realities of death even by 'well-informed' students. Fairly uniformly, they see themselves as dying suddenly and instantly in advanced age, probably of a coronary thrombosis. Another useful provocative technique described by Shneidman and others (Shneidman, 1972; Preston, 1973), is to invite participants to compose their own obituary.

Other sessions made use of role-play; in one instance to explore situations involving communication with a dying patient and her family; in another instance, while dealing with ethical problems regarding death, a group role-played a committee choosing which five out of 12 cases of terminal renal failure would be given places on a dialysis programme.

Following the large group sessions and meeting at least once a week, but as often and for as long as they wished, were small group sessions. Small multidisciplinary groups were set up, each with a group leader from different disciplines, but sharing some skills in facilitating group function. The content of group discussion was deliberately unstructured, although every week each group received a resource package to aid their studies. Such packages contained selective bibliographies and reprints of outstanding articles on the week's topic and a variety of other materials that could serve as a basis for discussion or study.

One problem has been encountered in many courses. Students are usually keen to meet and deal with real dying patients, to improve their skills at interviewing and helping. Patients generally seem to appreciate the interest and company this provides. But if many clinicians feel rather threatened by the establishment of discussion and teaching about death (and this certainly seems to be the case), then they are often especially reluctant to allow students access to their patients. More than one teacher has remarked, 'As soon as we start a course, there are no dying patients in the hospital'.

To help improve this situation, we developed a series of programmed and simulated patients; based on the method originated by Barrows (1971). These are perfectly fit volunteer members of the general public trained to simulate all the relevant features of real patients. They are strikingly convincing and genuine and among their advantages are that they can offer very comparable experiences to a sequence of student interviewers who can compare the effects of their differing techniques and abilities by direct observation through one-way mirrors, or by videotape review. The simulations we developed included a pathological grief reaction in a young widow, a teenager dying of leukaemia, an old man who approached death with impressive calmness and a middle-aged nurse who acknowledged that she had cancer but engaged in a protracted series of attempts to find a magical cure by visiting different famous hospitals.

We have found several other teaching aids particularly useful. There are numerous films now available, of which we found the following especially effective: *Until I Die* (Video-Nursing, Inc., Chicago) about the work of Elizabeth Kubler-Ross; *How Could I Not Be Among You?*, a film about the young American poet Ted Rosenthal, dying of leukaemia; and '*What Happened to the Pity?*', a fine BBC-TV documentary about the aftermath of the Aberfan disaster, a very moving study of responses to bereavement. On page 105 are listed some of the books we have found especially valuable in teaching and resources. Two of the finest are major works of literature: *The Death of Ivan Illych* by Leo Tolstoy, and *A Very Easy Death* by Simone de Beauvoir.

In closing, I quote from two dying people. First, the words of a student nurse in a poem that has been circulated to various nursing journals:

Death may get to be a routine to you, but it's new to me;
You may not see me as unique, but I have never died before;
To me, once is pretty unique.

Lastly, the words of a woman doctor who has written to me frequently, since she saw some of my work on a television programme, to share the experience of her slow and painful death with those I teach:

'When one is dying, there is a clarity of the true/false. Lack of sincerity is so obvious, it is cruel. While one must not wallow in grief, be genuinely kind and show that you care. I need encouragement and a cheerful, gentle few minutes—not hurried, not protracted. Don't make me feel I'm a bother, taking up time that could be put to better use. By all means say "Hi there, Mrs. Smith—I'll be along later": but keep that promise. Make me feel useful, perhaps asking my advice, using even a fragment from me; ask my opinion, find out my interests and mention them. Call me by name; I try to maintain my self-respect, and sometimes only my name may be left.

The relentless falling-off of visitors hurts so much. I'm not good company now, so I'm not wanted, and I cannot but feel bitter and childishly resentful. I feel that I need to cling to anybody, like a hurt child. All I ask is a little company, kindness, any indication that I am not forgotten. And useful. Let us know, till the end, that we are *loved*—in the true sense—that lessens pain. Heartbreak is much harder than the Heart Failure.'

REFERENCES

Barrows, H. S. (1971) *Simulated Patients*. Springfield, Ill: C. C. Thomas.

Barton, D. (1972) The need for including instruction on death and dying in the medical curriculum. *Journal of Medical Education*, **47**, 169.

Barton, D., Flexner, J. M., Van Eys, J. and Scott, C. E. (1972) Death and dying: a course for medical students. *Journal of Medical Education*, **47**, 945.

Feifel, H. *et al.* (1967) *Physicians Consider Death*. Proceedings of the Seventy-fifth Annual Convention, American Psychological Association.

Fulton, R. (Ed.) (1965) *Death and Identity*. New York: John Wiley.

Fulton, R. (Compiler) (1973) *A Bibliography on Death, Grief and Bereavement, 1845–1973* (3rd edition). Centre for Death Education and Research, University of Minnesota.

Knutson, A. L. (1968) Unpublished findings, cited in Brim, O. G. *et al.* (1970) *The Dying Patient*, p. 49. New York: Russell Sage Foundation.

Liston, E. H. (1973) Education on death and dying: a survey of American medical schools. *Journal of Medical Education*, **48**, 577.

Liston, E. H. (1974) Psychiatric aspects of life-threatening illness: a course for medical students. *International Journal of Psychiatry in Medicine*, **8**, No. 1, 51.

Olin, H. S. (1972) A proposed model to teach medical students the care of the dying patient. *Journal of Medical Education*, **47**, 564.

Preston, C. E. (1973) Behavior modification: a therapeutic approach to ageing and dying. *Postgraduate Medicine*, **54**, No. 6, 64.

Sabatini, P. and Kastenbaum, R. (1973) The do-it-yourself death certificate as a research technique. *Life-Threatening Behavior*, **3**, No. 1, 51.

Saul, E. V. and Kass, J. S. (1969) Study of anticipated anxiety in a medical school setting. *Journal of Medical Education*, **44**, 526.

Schoenberg, B. and Carr, A. C. (1972) Educating the health professional in the psychosocial care of the terminally ill, in *Psychosocial Aspects of Terminal Care* (Eds. Schoenberg, B., Carr, A. C., Peretz, D. and Kutscher, A. H.), pp. 3–15. New York: Columbia University Press.

Shneidman, E. S. (1972) Can a young person write his own obituary? *Life-Threatening Behavior*, **2**, No. 4, 262.

Simpson, M. A. (1973a) Teaching about death and dying. *Nursing Times*, **69**, No. 13, 442.

Simpson, M. A. (1973b) *Teaching on Death and Dying to Medical and Para-medical Students*. Proceedings: ASME Scientific Meeting, London, February, 1973.

Simpson, M. A. (1974) *The Do-It-Yourself Death Certificate in Teaching about Death and Dying*. Presented to the ACMC Scientific Meeting, Calgary, 1974. (In press.)

Simpson, M. A. (1975) Teaching about Death and Dying in British Medical Schools. (In press.)

BIBLIOGRAPHY

Helping Children Learn about Death

Arnstein, Helene S. (1962) *What to Tell your Child about Birth, Illness, Death, Divorce and Other Family Crises.* Indianapolis: Bobbs-Merrill.

Best, Pauline (1948) An experience in interpreting death to children. *Journal of Pastoral Care,* **2,** 29.

Grollman, Earl A. (Ed.) (1967) *Explaining Death to Children.* Boston: Beacon Press.

Grollman, Earl A. (1970) *Talking about Death.* A Dialogue Between Parent and Child, p. 32. Boston: Beacon Press.

Jackson, E. N. (1965) *Telling a Child about Death.* New York: Channel Press.

Lasker, A. A. (1972) Telling children the facts of death. *Your Child,* Winter, p. 1.

Lichtenwalner, M. E. (1964) Children ask about death. *International Journal of Religious Education,* **40,** 14.

Mahler, M. S. (1950) Helping children to accept death. *Child Study,* **27,** 98.

Reed, E. L. (1970) *Helping Children with the Mystery of Death.* Nashville: Abingdon Press.

Wolf, A. W. M. (1958 & 1973) *Helping Your Child to Understand Death.* New York: Child Study Press.

Adult and Professional Education about Death

Farmer, J. A. (1970) Death education: adult education in the face of a taboo. *Omega,* **1,** 109.

Kubler-Ross, Elizabeth (1970) *On Death and Dying.* London: Tavistock Publications and New York: Macmillan.

Kubler-Ross, Elizabeth (1972) Facing up to death. *Today's Education,* **61,** 30.

Leviton, D. (1972) A course on death education and suicide prevention: implications for health education. *Journal of the American College Health Association,* **19,** 217.

Leviton, D. (1971) Death, bereavement and suicide education, in *New Directions in Health Education* (Ed. Read, D. A.). New York: Macmillan.

Leviton, D. (1969) The need for education on death and suicide. *Journal of School Health,* **39,** 270.

Morgan, E. (Ed.) (1973) *A Manual of Death Education and Simple Burial.* Burnsville, North Carolina: The Celo Press.

Park, Roswell (1912) Thanatology: a questionnaire and a plea for a neglected study. *Journal of the American Medical Association,* **58,** 1243.

Peniston, D. H. (1962) The importance of death education in family life. *Family Life Coordinator,* **11,** 15.

Scott, F. G. and Brewer, R. M. (Eds.) (1971) *Confrontations of Death: A Book of Readings and a Suggested Method of Instruction.* Corvallis, Oregon: Continuing Education Publications.

Somerville, R. M. (1971) Death education as part of family life education. *The Family Coordinator,* **20,** 209.

White, D. K. (1970) An undergraduate course in death. *Omega,* **1,** 167.

FURTHER READING

Fiction and Literature

Agee, James (1971) *A Death in the Family.* London: P. Owen.

Alvarez, A. (1971) *The Savage God.* London: Weidenfeld & Nicolson.

De Beauvoir, Simone (1966) *A Very Easy Death*. London: Deutsch and Weidenfeld & Nicolson.
Gunther, John (1949) *Death Be Not Proud*. New York: Harper & Row.
Plath, Sylvia (1967) *The Bell Jar*. London: Faber & Faber.
Rosenthal, Ted (1973) *How Could I Not Be Among You?* New York: Braziller.
Tolstoy, Leo (1971) *The Death of Ivan Illych*. London: Oxford University Press.
Trumbo, Dalton (1967) *Johnny Got His Gun*. London: Corgi Books.
Waugh, Evelyn (1965) *The Loved One*. London: Chapman & Hall.

Medical and Professional
Choron, Jacques (1963) *Death and Western Thought*. London: Collier-Macmillan.
Choron, Jacques (1964) *Death and Modern Man*. London: Collier-Macmillan.
Feifel, H. (Ed.) (1959) *The Meaning of Death*. New York: McGraw-Hill.
Kastenbaum, R. and Aisenburg, R. (1972) *Psychology of Death*. New York: Springer Publishing Co. Inc.
Kubler-Ross, Elizabeth (1970) *On Death and Dying*. London: Tavistock Publications and New York: Macmillan.
Mitford, Jessica (1963) *The American Way of Death*. Greenwich, CT: Fawcett.
Parkes, Colin Murray (1972) *Bereavement*. London: Tavistock Publications.
Schoenberg, B., Carr, A. C., Peretz, D. and Kutscher, A. H. (Eds.) (1970) *Loss and Grief: Psychological Management in Medical Practice*. New York: Columbia University Press.
Shneidman, E. (1972) *The Deaths of Man*. New York: Quadrangle/New York Times.
Sudnow, David (1967) *Passing On: The Social Organization of Dying*. Englewood Cliffs, NJ: Prentice-Hall.
Weisman, Avery (1972) *On Dying and Denying*. New York: Behavioral Publications.

10

Pastoral Care

NORMAN AUTTON

> *Dying is normal—a healthy thing to do—*
> *everyone does it.*
>
> R. Lamerton

> *Beside the bed where parting life was laid,*
> *And sorrow, guilt and pain by turns dismayed,*
> *The reverend champion stood. At his control*
> *Despair and anguish fled the struggling soul;*
> *Comfort came down the trembling wretch to raise,*
> *And his last faltering accents whispered praise.*
>
> Oliver Goldsmith, 'The Deserted Village'

> *God be at mine end, and at my departing.*
>
> Old Sarum Primer

THERE IS OFTEN a sense of awe and uneasiness surrounding the bedside of the dying, and no matter how experienced doctor and chaplain might be, or how often they have seen men die, the drama of death itself never seems to cease to be grievous and disquieting. In his *Thoughts for the Times on War and Death*, Freud points out that

> '. . . in the unconscious every one of us is convinced of his own immortality. As to the death of another, the civilised man will carefully avoid speaking of such a possibility in the hearing of the person concerned . . . our habit is to lay stress on the fortuitous causation of the death—accident, disease, infection, advanced age; in this way we betray our endeavour to modify the significance of death from a necessity to an accident.'

We are apt to amend the words of the Psalmist and cry that although 'a thousand shall fall beside me, and ten thousand at my right hand, it shall not come nigh *me*!'

Our own personal feelings, therefore, need to be closely watched. Unless we are reconciled to dying and have come to terms with death ourselves we shall always be tempted to avoid a meaningful relationship with the terminally ill patient.

Our own anxiety and inhibitions will impede and interfere so that we do not hear what is being said to us. We shall misinterpret what is told us and there will be an insecure ring about the words we use, giving reassurances which cannot be substantiated, offering theological sermonettes which, while probably true, are irrelevant at that particular time to the person who confronts us with his need.

Each death bed can be a stark reminder of our own mortality and death, for John Donne's words still ring true. 'Any man's death diminishes me, because I am involved in Mankind; And therefore never send to know for whom the bell tolls; It tolls for thee.'

When we have put our own house in order we can then be truly available and sensitively responsive to the various needs of those to whom we minister. We shall be better equipped to deal with the other's feelings, thoughts, hopes and aspirations, and even his doubt and despair, all of which are important and need to be shared.

SPIRITUAL NEEDS

Pastoral care of the dying is primarily concerned not with physical symptoms but with a spiritual unity which is conducive to wholeness of being. The understanding of the spiritual dimension of the patient sheds much insight upon his total health. We live in an age when the quantity of life seems more important than its quality; when health and longevity have been so highly prized that those who are being deprived of them are left in an emotional chaos and a spiritual vacuum. Faith is held out to the patient not as an escape but as an inner courage and inspiration to face up to what cannot be escaped.

Some terminally ill patients overwhelmed, as often they are, with fear and loneliness wish to discuss spiritual concerns in order to resolve some of their feelings of isolation. Others, being aware of the shortness of their days, seek solace in pastoral and priestly ministrations to help them put their affairs, material and spiritual, in order. Many seem to have no religious beliefs at all and face out the inevitable with a 'grin and bear it' approach. Each attitude has to be respected; each need met.

Spiritual care can mediate a healthy acceptance of the situation as it is, free from false hopes and shallow reassurances. There will be no place for playing on feelings of guilt; no attempt to erect barriers of communication with pious clichés and ritualistic reasonings, for these merely threaten and abort any significant relationship between chaplain and patient.

It is not for the chaplain to discuss the medical chances of survival, which is the task of the doctor. It is, however, his function to *relate*, to *accept* and to *listen*. In this way he will be able to diagnose some of the basic fears uppermost in the patient's mind. He will pay far more attention to feelings rather than words, watching with gentleness and listening with attention and respect. He can be asking himself such questions about some of the spiritual and emotional needs of the patient. 'Who is this person to whom I am ministering?' 'How is he responding to his present predicament?' 'What are some of his special spiritual needs at this time?' The chaplain, in recognising some of the feelings and demands of the sufferer, can then help him to *absorb*, *interpret* and *transcend* them, so that the temporal eventually becomes transformed into the eternal.

What are some of the fears most frequently encountered in those who are dying? Any clear-cut classifications can of course be misleading, for each patient must be seen as a unique individual. It is sometimes assumed that the Christian patient should not have any fears of death at all, and consequently a sense of guilt can often be fostered where this belief has been firmly held. But a fear of death is both normal and natural as well as universal. St Augustine in his work *On the Gospel of St John* asks, 'Ought the mind of the Christian to be troubled even at the prospect of death?' and replies:

'Strong-minded, indeed, are those Christians, if such there are, who experience no trouble at all in the prospect of death; but for all that, are they stronger-minded than Christ? Who would have the madness to say so? And what else, then, does His being troubled signify, but that, by voluntarily assuming the likeness of their weakness, He comforted the weak members in His body, that is in His Church; to the end that, if any of His own are still troubled at the approach of death, they may fix their gaze upon Him, and so be kept from thinking themselves castaways on this account, and being swallowed up in the more grievous death of despair?'

The fear to be avoided is that which has no hope or assurance; the fear that cankers and destroys spiritual strength and resources and leads only to despair and decay. Personal sanctity is no panacea against the fears of death, but what the Christian patient knows is that for him the real 'sting' of death has been removed. 'Yea, though I walk through the valley of the shadow of death, I will fear no evil . . .' (Ps. 23: 4).

There is often fear of the unknown, for the hereafter is 'an undiscovered country from whose bourne no traveller returns'; fear of regression, pain, loss of family and friends, one's own identity, or self-control. Fears of loneliness and abandonment are also very commonly encountered, for each of us must die alone. We are reminded by Paul Tillich that '. . . there is the ultimate loneliness of having to die. In the anticipation of our death we remain alone. No communication with others can remedy it, as no other's presence in the actual hour of our dying can conceal the fact that it is our death and our death alone. In the hour of death we are cut off from the whole universe and everything in it. We are deprived of things and beings which made us forget our being alone. Who can endure this loneliness?' Yes, who indeed! One of the basic elements of pastoral care will therefore be that of companionship, supporting the patient with *faith, friendship* and *fellowship*. The doctor and nurse will have other patients to tend; the ward routine has to continue. The chaplain is often the only person who has the time to stay alongside the patient and his family. He symbolises, 'I am with you. You are not alone.' Once with the patient, the chaplain's person, his physical presence, is often his most significant ministry; some of his deepest teachings will be non-verbal.

Such an attitude is well summed up by Dr Cicely Saunders, Medical Director of St Christopher's Hospice, Sydenham.

'They [the dying] need more than sympathy and sedatives. They need something that was summed up for us for all time with the words "Watch with me". I think that phrase means persevering with the practical and developing the many skills that can help. But I think above all it means listening without necessarily knowing the answers. It means "Do not forget to be simple" and "Be prepared just to be there". We must somehow say to these people, "You matter because you are you", and give everything that will enable the patient to live up until he dies and the family to go on living afterwards' (Saunders, 1972).

RELIGIOUS BELIEFS

Do the religious beliefs of a patient influence the way in which he faces up to terminal illness? Dr Kubler-Ross (1970), in her researches and work with the dying, found that, on the whole, religious patients seemed to differ very little in their attitude from those without a religion. The truly religious patient with an intrinsic faith, however, was helped to face up to his illness. Professor Hinton (1967) reached similar conclusions:

'Although many religious people find comfort concerning death through their faith, not all with religious beliefs are reassured. It was even found in one study that those with religious beliefs had more fears of death than the non-religious . . . Those who had firm religious faith and attended their church weekly or frequently were most free from anxiety . . . the tepid believers, who professed faith but made little outward observance of it, were most anxious to a significant extent.'

Faith, when firmly and confidently held and observed, provides courage and hope rather than doubt and despair. It is worth observing that agnostics seem to be as free from anxiety as regular churchgoers. 'Lukewarm' Christian patients seem to experience the greatest degree of fear and anxiety. Those who have made sense of life seem more able to make sense of death. The stable personality is more able to deal with the stresses and strains of dying, and seems to derive comfort and strength from his beliefs.

TO TELL OR NOT TO TELL

There can be no hard and fast rules, no clear-cut answers to the problem of telling or withholding the truth from the patient, for each is a unique individual in a unique situation. There are some patients who are strong-minded whilst others are over-sensitive. A number of patients seem to sense their true condition and its prognosis, whilst some are prepared to accept the diagnosis but deny the prognosis. There are, however, probably far more patients than we sometimes realise who would prefer to know the truth. A nagging fear, together with a dwindling hope, is often far harder to bear than the thought of impending death. Fear of the unknown is sometimes more difficult to bear than fear of the known. A conspiracy of silence results, in many instances, in inhibition and deceit all round, and such uneasiness and tension tend to make the patient more anxious, resentful and full of self-pity. Confidence in the relationship of doctor and patient can soon be broken and the game of pretence lost. The medical world is sometimes prone to justify its silence on humanitarian grounds, that it is kinder for the patient not to know the truth. In some instances this silence can be a mere rationalisation of the doctor's inability to face up to the fact of death himself, and consequently the easier and simpler course of avoidance is carried through.

Some patients often have far more moral and spiritual courage to face up to death than is realised by those who are ministering to them. It should never be right to tell deliberate lies, for each patient has the right to know and to learn the true facts about his condition, should he so desire. Often it is difficult to glean what the patient really wants to know. Rarely is the question put bluntly, 'Am I going to die?' If asked at all it is often put the other way round: 'Am I going to get better, doctor?' Some prefer not to ask questions or receive explicit answers. Although they may be aware of their true state, they seek protection through silence and suppression. There are others again who seem to deny or distort the truth to their own advantage.

When the truth is to be given it should be imparted with grace and dignity. 'Glib answers no one has', writes Gerald J. Aronson, 'but I think we must be guided by the principle of permitting and helping the patient to keep up as much as possible *the role that is important to him.*' To fulfil this adequately four general rules are suggested:

1. Do not tell the patient anything which might induce psycho-pathology. One is guided here, he suggests, by the clinical feel and the response of the patient to our comment and manner as we slowly go along with him in the course of his illness.
2. Hope must never die too far ahead of the patient.
3. The gravity of the situation should not be minimised . . . the patient will not fail to understand from our demeanour that his situation is serious . . . more good deaths are spoiled because the physician tries to jolly the patient or neglect him as a sentient being.
4. Telling the patient about his impending death in such a way as to avoid just idly sitting around, awaiting death. We must try to estimate the duration of a man's psychological present.

What is needed of the pastoral care of both doctor and chaplain at this time is *sympathetic communication.* So often relationship speaks louder than words. Often, too, the dying tell us rather than we them. What matters most is not what is told but *how* it is told. 'Personally I think that a quiet straight answer with a clear look in the eye is as a rule the best reply,' suggests W. N. Leak, 'and it is usually answered by a quiet "Thank you, doctor", or "I knew it". It is vastly easier to manage the patient after such a simple and sincere acknowledgement of the fact. And if the doctor can honestly also speak of that land where ". . . there shall be no more death neither sorrow nor crying, neither shall there be any more pain . . ." the last dying days may be full of hope and peace instead of violent struggle and despair.'

If we are perspective and sensitive to the needs of our patients; if we have been prepared to watch with them at the bedside and not hasten away in retreat, we shall be better equipped to gain that sensitivity to understand and appreciate their true feelings and thoughts, and so help them die in dignity and peace.

On the one hand we shall help those who so wish to express verbally their deepest longings and innermost needs and, on the other hand, respect the feelings of those who wish to remain silent and not have the true facts disclosed to them. Our whole approach will need much tact, skill and patience. So much will depend on our reflection to such questions as: Who is this patient? What is his temperament? What are the circumstances that might make the imparting of this information rightful?

LISTENING TO THE DYING

So often our most important role is a passive one, listening and being alert to cues in the conversation which tell us about the real *person of the patient*. Listening can express the fullest of sympathy and the deepest of understanding, enabling, as it does, the chaplain or doctor, to share the unresolved problems and conflicting emotions of the patient. To love the dying we must listen with *feeling*, *understanding* and *acceptance*; not merely in a cosy friendly way but on occasions in a competent and professional attitude. The experienced chaplain will listen to the feelings of the dying, not only to what is said but also to what is not said, for the latter is often far more significant than the former. In this way he is listening to what the patient is really wanting to say. Such creative silence at the bedside helps the patient grope for values that transcend both health and survival; to offer up his whole being in a faith that encompasses even his pain and his death. In such a climate, too, the truth can be spoken in an openness to reality; health seems not to be the ultimate end of life after all, and death not the worst thing that can happen to a man.

Many who minister to the needs of the dying will be able to re-echo some words of Dr Kubler-Ross (1970), 'Those who have the strength and the love to sit with a dying patient in *the silence that goes beyond words* will know that this moment is neither frightening nor painful, but a peaceful cessation of the functioning of the body.'

PHYSICAL TOUCH

Terminal illness often creates a deep sense of disintegration with its accompanying anxiety and insecurity, and physical contact can be of much support. To hold on to an outstretched hand in loneliness and pain provides a sense of attachment, reassurance and comfort. It is an outward and tangible sign of an inward acceptance. It is an act which can mean far more than words. As one patient put it, 'I remember very little of what was happening about me, but the two things which seemed to give me reassurance was the voice of the chaplain and the feel of his hand in mine.'

We must be mindful of the fact that hearing is the last of the senses to go, and so heed what is said in the presence of dying persons. A patient in the midst of a rather distressful illness may see himself as 'abhorrent' or 'untouchable', and physical contact does much to calm such an attitude of mind, bridging as it does the chasm between the living and the dead.

THE MINISTRY OF THE CHAPLAIN

Teamwork

In attempting to meet the needs of the dying, both doctor and chaplain, together with other members of the healing team, soon realise that many of the problems involved are larger than any one professional discipline can resolve in isolation. Each needs the support of the other; each needs the humility to learn from the other. At the bedside of the dying both church and medicine should stand complementary one to the other, with no clear-cut lines of demarcation—'the body for the doctor, the soul for the priest!' It surely cannot be right to adopt such an over-simplified distinction for both are inseparable, and doctor and chaplain are together tending one and the same person in the bed—the doctor's patient, the clergyman's parishioner, God's creation. Indeed the late Lord Fisher of Lambeth once went so far as to say that, '. . . when it comes to dying, there is no distinction between doctor and chaplain—both are pastors, and the faith of the doctor can often do far more than that of the chaplain, just because the doctor has been fighting the battle of life and death with the patient day by day more intimately than can often be the case for the chaplain.' Worcester, too, seemed to bear this out when he wrote that, '. . . the dying do not always recognise the difference between the clerical and medical professions. They seem also unable to recognise the difference between the need for physical relief and that of consolation.'

It is of the utmost importance that the chaplain be fully recognised by and taken into the confidence of the other members of the team, for otherwise his ministry becomes stultified and he himself frustrated.

Preparation

Ideally, a relationship should have been fostered with the terminal patient long before his illness becomes severe. A stranger, be he either doctor or chaplain, arriving on the scene in the final stages of an illness can be not only disturbing but disrupting to the patient's peace of mind. Commenting on the difficulty of confronting the terminally ill patient when there has been lack of earlier preparation, Dr Paul Tournier confesses,

> 'I have always felt that my fault lay further back . . . in not having been able earlier, when the patient was not so near death, to establish close contact with him and to create that climate of spiritual fellowship without which the truth cannot be told. It is in speaking of the meaning of things that we enter into this fellowship giving the patient an opportunity of talking to us about the things that are weighing on his mind, long before he has reached the last extremity.'

Far too frequently the chaplain is not summoned until almost all is over.

There is need, too, for continuity of care. The person with whom the patient is best able to communicate should not withdraw, but be prepared to stay and relate. 'My friends and family do not know what to say to me now that they know that I know', remarked one patient, 'but I can speak freely to the chaplain.' The person to whom the patient can best relate in his crisis must be prepared to stay.

Prayer and Sacrament

Counselling, prayer, bible-reading, the sacraments, all play a part where they are appropriate and meaningful to the patient. Where there is a prayerful relationship, the sacraments become a vital part of the chaplain's ministrations, for then they have a meaning to the patient as well as to himself. It will be necessary to adapt methods of approach to meet the particular spiritual needs of each individual patient. Some will be familiar with the teaching of their respective church, and here spiritual care can be direct and devotional. Others may be nominal or lapsed members, and some of no religious persuasion at all.

The approach of the chaplain will in part depend upon the particular denomination and liturgical background of the patient,

which he will do well to respect. His aim will be to help the terminally ill patient see more and more of God's love for him, and
where desirable the patient can be led to acts of penitence, prayer
and self-oblation. The sacrament of penance will assure him of
forgiveness, holy unction or anointing of the sick will sustain and
strengthen him, the sacrament of Holy Communion will be his
'viaticum', and commendatory prayers will commit him into
God's hands. In those instances where there is little or no
allegiance to the Christian faith the very integrity of the chaplain's
presence and companionship, as well as those of the other
members of the team, will often be sufficient, for such love and
respect are all part of the Christian message. In this way there is
a sense of community and genuine fellowship—qualities so surely
needed to combat an institutionalised and professionalised mode
of dying. If the dying can be helped to realise the presence of God
then their pain and suffering can be used and transformed.

Orthodox Jews are ministered to by the local Rabbi who will
read from the Jewish rites. After death the body may be removed
to the mortuary, but the washings can only be performed by
members of the Jewish Burial Society.

It is important, too, that the spiritual needs of immigrants be
adequately met. Moslems have very strict rules and are usually
told they are going to die. They are expected to confess their sins
and seek forgiveness. The body, after death and the washings, will
face Mecca, and no one other than friends and family must move
it. Hindus, too, are strict about who should touch the body after
death. A thread is usually tied around the patient's wrist or neck
to symbolise a blessing, and this remains *in situ* after death.
Buddhists have the Sutras recited together with a blessing. A
picture of Buddha is normally brought to the bedside, so that the
patient can have a happy death.

Whatever the religious observances might be, they all lay a
great responsibility on the priest or minister.

'How great, how solemn, how awful an undertaking! To
accompany to the very brink of that dark river a dying man,
to whom all is necessarily strange . . . to guide the steps of the
soul towards that plunge into the invisible . . . who is sufficient
for these things? . . . What earnestness should we feel, not to be
found helplessly silent or shamefully formal in the necessary

suggestions of last words, last consolations, last prayers, to the dying. What manner of persons, I repeat, ought we pastors to be—were it but for this last cause—in all holy conversation and godliness' (Williams, 1960).

LEARNING FROM THE DYING

Finally, in pastoral care of the dying, we who are members of the helping and healing team must always be aware of the ways in which they can in turn minister to us. We must always be alert to the lessons they can teach us, for it is only the dying who are in the position of showing how best the dying can be helped and cared for. We shall very soon discover there is a mutuality of ministry. Indeed there are many times when our roles become reversed—the patient becomes the 'chaplain' ministering and teaching us. And how many lessons there are to be learned! They are our teachers, and we shall all do well to share the last chapter of their personal pilgrimage through the valley of the shadow of death, reflecting on the significance of those experiences for a clearer understanding of ourselves as persons, and our respective roles as chaplains and doctors.

REFERENCES

Aronson, G. J. (1959) *The Meaning of Death* (Ed. Feifel, H.), p. 252. New York: McGraw-Hill.
Hinton, J. (1967) *Dying*, pp. 37 and 83. Harmondsworth: Penguin Books.
Kubler-Ross, Elizabeth (1970) *On Death and Dying*, p. 237. London: Tavistock Publications.
Kubler-Ross, Elizabeth (1970) ibid. p. 246.
Leak, W. N. (1948) *Practitioner* (August).
Saunders, Cicely (1972) In *Care of the Dying*. DHSS Reports, No. 5. London: HMSO, 1973.
Tournier, P. (1954) *A Doctor's Casebook in the Light of the Bible*. London: SCM Press.
Williams, R. R. (Ed.) (1960) *The World of Life*, pp. 101-2. London: SPCK.
Worcester (1960) *Care of the Aged, the Dying and the Dead*. Springfield, Ill: C. C. Thomas.

11

The Care of the Bereaved

J. R. CASSWELL

THE FACT that a chapter, even though a brief one, with such a title should be included in this handbook intended for many readers, including medical students, is a welcome indication of the wide connotation that is being given to the subject of 'medical care' these days. How far the busy medical practitioner will be able to fit it in with the increasing demands made upon his time, and patience, under the National Health Service is problematical. It really carries us back to the old concept of the 'family doctor', so that the doctor's 'care' becomes analogous to the clerical 'cure' of souls; indeed the two words are identical etymologically.

The effective exercise of this care will require a strong sense of vocation, and approaches the realm in which 'doctors are born, not made', though doubtless, even those who are by nature comparatively insensitive will, by frequent contact with suffering and sorrow, develop in some measure the qualities of understanding and sympathy which this ministry will require.

The doctor who wishes to exercise this kind of care will see it, no doubt, as related to both psychological medicine and social medicine; the latter when the bereaved individual is old or infirm, lonely, or impoverished by the bereavement.

It will be well to consider the matter first from the standpoint of psychological medicine, as this will cover all cases, whether there is consequent social need or not.

It is, perhaps, most helpful to regard bereavement as an amputation. It is a trauma in the realm of the affections and emotions analogous to the loss of a limb in the physical realm, in fact to the loss of more than a limb. Catullus wrote of the lady of his affections as 'the half of my life', and many a husband and wife has felt that more than a half of life has been taken when the other partner has been removed by death. Just as when a limb is amputated the patient will continue to feel 'ghost' pains in the limb that is no longer there, and will require physiotherapy to learn how to live without it, so will the bereaved individual, or family, feel ghost pains in the emotions and affections. These are far harder to bear, where the bond of affection has been real and deep, than are physical 'ghost' pains. They may last a very long time, for some commentators think that Jacob never got over Rachel's death, and therapy will be needed to bring about adjustment to living without the one who has been lost.

This, then, is the position with which the doctor is faced, and if he is to deal with it effectually it will tax all his own resources of inner strength, as well as of time. The greatest source of comfort will be the 'consolations' not of philosophy, David Hume's mother discovered *that* when she sought it from her son, but of strong spiritual faith. If the doctor has a personal experience of 'the God of all comfort' and can communicate it in any way to his bereaved patient he will be doing an immense service. But even where this is not the case, the doctor, as a result both of training and experience, may be expected to be a person of quick perception and deep understanding of human nature. When all that has been acquired in this way is brought to bear on the individual case in hand the doctor should be able to impart solid comfort and encouragement. Sympathy can be conveyed by a glance, a slight pressure of the hand on arm or shoulder, or a brief word of understanding. This will provide just the right (occasional) stimulus to the revival of hope, enabling the bereaved individual to pick up the broken threads of life that seem to have been severed by death. Sympathy, however, should not be overdone, or it will have the effect of turning the patient in upon himself, something to be avoided at all costs. The aim must be, just as in the case of those who have suffered an amputation, to enable the patient to walk alone. On the other hand, the hearty back-slapping 'cheer up' approach is worse than useless and may be positively harmful: 'As vinegar upon nitre so is he that singeth songs to a heavy heart.' But it is a good maxim never to encourage people to feel sorry for themselves, however painful their lot.

If the doctor knows the family well, a word of appreciation of the qualities of the one they have lost will have a tonic effect in enabling them to realise that others besides themselves hold their dear one in high regard, and that the life that has now come to an end has not been lived in vain, but has made its contribution, however small, to the well-being not only of the family, but also of the community. This, of course, will not apply in anything like the same measure in the case of the death of a very young child, but in at least one such case, Bishop Taylor Smith, a former Chaplain-General to the Forces, pointed out to the sorrowing parents that when a shepherd wants to get his flock into the fold, he sometimes has to pick up one of the lambs and carry it into the fold first that the others may follow.

To turn to that aspect of the care of the bereaved that relates to social medicine, it will be obvious that where bereavement has left a partner already advanced in years to face the future alone, very real problems can arise. Most of us are made for companionship, and loneliness, even when not caused by recent bereavement, can itself be a grievous burden, but this is greatly aggravated when to it is added the sorrow of separation caused by death. Discrimination will, however, need to be exercised in any efforts to provide companionship for the lonely. For people to find satisfaction in each other's society, there needs to be not only some degree of community of interests but also some measure of affinity of temperament and outlook. To say that no one aged over seventy should be allowed to live alone may be a rash dictum, and it would produce no benefit to bereaved and lonely people to compel them into close association with others of entirely different ways of thought and conduct. The doctor will know what facilities for meeting others, or even for living with others, are available, and his wisdom will be to seek to promote contacts, whether occasional or permanent, with those whose society will be agreeable and stimulating to his patients, and to whom the patients themselves will be able to make some worthwhile contribution. The object of such contacts will be to rehabilitate bereaved individuals, both psychologically and emotionally, and they may need to be warned not to talk too much of their own private griefs, or of the virtues of the one whose loss they are mourning. The maxim 'Laugh and the world laughs with you, weep and you weep alone', may seem to the sorrowing individual to be lacking in sympathy, but, for good or ill, it is largely true.

When to the sorrows of bereavement and consequent loneliness are added those of infirmity, or even incapacity, the problem becomes acute. The bereaved patient at times will feel an almost overwhelming sense of desolation, and much wise sympathy and patient understanding will be called for, as well as the more practical aids that may be provided by community services where such aids are not available by private or family arrangement.

Fortunately, in these days, bereavement will rarely, if ever, result in complete financial destitution. Should it do so, the solution to this aspect of the problem is really outside the doctor's hands, though he will need to know what assistance, both public and private, is available, and to use great tact in urging his patient to make use of it. Quite often, however, where there is no absolute destitution, there may be a sudden and serious decline in living standards. This may involve such re-adjustments as moving into a smaller house, giving up a car, or removing children from a fee-paying school. It is not always possible to effect these changes immediately, or even quickly. People faced with such problems are, in these days, likely to look to the doctor for comfort and support as well as for advice, whereas in previous generations they would have looked to the vicar or minister. The doctor will, indeed, need to be a person of ready sympathy and deep wisdom to deal not only with the mechanics of such a situation, but also with the living, sentient human beings who find themselves thus placed.

In the psychological aspect of the care of the bereaved, then, the personality of the doctor will be a factor of great importance, and well will it be for the bereaved individual or family if the doctor has the 'human touch'. It will be a great advantage, too, if he can offer helpful suggestions for reading, whether on the highest spiritual level, or on the merely practical level, such as is offered to chest and heart patients by the magazine *Hope* of the Chest and Heart Association.

On the social level the doctor will best care for the bereaved by keeping himself informed of the various associations, both statutory and voluntary, that are available to meet all the differing needs to which bereavement gives rise. As these associations are likely to be continually increasing, fairly constant effort may be needed to keep abreast of developments in this field.

What has been written can, perhaps, be summed up by reminding the doctor that in the care of the bereaved, as in so many other departments of life, character is at least as important

E

as professional knowledge and skill. What is needed on the psychological level is the warm, human sympathy that will enable the doctor to enter into the thoughts and feelings of those who have been bereaved—what the Americans call 'empathy'. On the social (or practical) side the doctor will need to give expression to that sympathy by ascertaining what are the practical needs of the individual or the family, and what State or private resources are available to meet them.

12

Practical Thoughts

A RELIGIOUS OF THE SOCIETY OF ST MARGARET
and
P. A. DOWNIE

> *Death has a hundred hands and walks by a thousand ways.*
>
> T. S. Eliot

IN DISCUSSING WORK with the dying one can only generalise, for
no two people will behave in the same way and each act of dying
is essentially individualistic. The practical approach to this subject
is set within the context of the Passion and Resurrection of Our
Lord, for the two authors firmly believe that the care of the dying
becomes more intelligible if seen in this way. This does not mean
that those of no faith cannot do this work, but it does imply that
there is a real need to see the full purpose of life in order to give
the necessary hope, reassurance and care as earthly life draws to
its close.

GENERAL PHILOSOPHY

It is sad that many nurses, medical students and others think of
the care of the dying as a specialty and, sadder still, that they
expect to find a textbook to tell them how to do it. Death is an
inevitable fact of life; indeed human existence within the time
sequence can be summed up in two words 'life' and 'death', and
they are the only two certainties common to us all, spanning an
unknown distance from the moment of conception to the point at
which earthly life is extinguished.

'Death is not merely an appendix to life in the manner of the
ending of a bad play that might turn out anyhow. Death is built
into life's structure and issues from its course. It is present long
before the conclusion, actually throughout the whole develop-

ment of life. Life has been defined as a moment directed towards death' (Guardini, 1954).

The care of the dying should therefore be seen as a part of the whole treatment plan for a patient.

Certainly death is the last part of human life, but for everything alive it is this last part which is most crucial; death brings man's life to its fulfilment for good or ill and the shape of that life will require a conclusion to give it final validity. Death remains a reality but equally it does become a gateway into a new life. Within this base reality there is a spirituality which can lift physical death to a higher plane and which gives the true purpose to all our lives. All our life we are steadily preparing for death and there is no doubt that the manner of a person's death is a reflection of the way he has lived; one of the very real practical aspects of this work in many cases is to help patients to live. For some indeed, the last few months may be the very first time that they have understood what living really means.

> Teach me to live, that I may dread
> The grave as little as my bed;
> Teach me to die, that so I may
> Rise glorious at the awful day![1]

Care of the dying cannot be neatly slotted into a definite period of time; the actual process of dying may be sudden or it may be a progressive decline, of failing faculties and functions. It is about the latter group that most of the practical comments will be made, since it is these patients who require the encouragement and reassurance to accept their weaknesses and to live. It is of these that the question, 'Should the patient be told of his approaching death?', will be asked. In general the answer is probably 'Yes', in as much as they are able to bear it. There is no need to be cold and dogmatic; rather sow the seed and then wait and see what follows. Certainly this telling should be done early in the care of patients so that they are able to assimilate the truth and to be helped to come to an understanding. This is one of the reasons why early admission to the Homes which specialise in the care of patients suffering from progressive illness, is so earnestly hoped for.

[1]Bishop T. Ken, 'Glory to Thee my God This night', Hymns A & M, Revised, 23, English Hymnal No. 267.

Patients suffering from progressive disease, and particularly those who may have been treated with cytotoxic drugs, become less and less able to respond to the demands of brain and body and consequently, they look always to the familiar things. How often does one see a distracted patient who on being asked what is wrong, will tell you that she has lost her handkerchief, her glasses or a special letter. It is the same reaction as that of the small child who cries at night because she has lost a favourite toy; find the missing article and all is well. It is not the slightest good telling either the dying patient or the child, not to worry; this is not acceptable. Peace of mind is essential and the nurse, or whoever is involved, will have to make the time to find and restore the focal object, and what is more, this must be done in a spirit of willingness and not impatience.

PRACTICAL OBSERVATIONS

Practical care for the dying patient demands the outward showing of all those qualities which should be inherent not only in nurses but in all who are involved in the healing professions. Nursing *per se* is not confined to caring for the living. It is an art to be used for the total care of man according to his needs and the care at the bedside of the dying patient is an essential facet of a nurse's work.

It is always difficult to determine when a patient begins to die. Many people suffering from chronic progressive illness may decline slowly over months and imperceptibly slip into that period which the skilled nurse instinctively recognises as preceding the act of dying. The yardstick of all care of the dying is to improve the quality of life remaining in the individual patient; it may entail keeping one patient drowsy and thus unaware of pain, whilst allowing another patient to live more actively and even more dangerously than would normally have been considered (Graeme, 1975).

It is essentially experience and even intuition which guides one in the right approach for each patient. Overall must be the desire to allow patients to live and this can entail carrying out strange requests. One of the authors vividly recalls having to break and enter a house for a dying patient who had mislaid the key to her newly acquired property and who was determined to survey the alterations which had been carried out. Similarly, strange requests for food and drink are not uncommon, and it can be worth more than any drug to fulfil such desires.

This is *not* the time to insist on special diets or treatments. This is the time to keep to a familiar pattern which can be understood and accepted by the patient. It is a time for compassion, for real understanding of a patient's needs and for being around to listen and support both patient and relatives. Sensible, simple answers should be given to questions and if an honest answer is not possible then say so—do not be tempted to hedge. Never must a dying patient be allowed to feel that nothing more can be done for him, or that he is no longer capable of taking family decisions. He needs to see people round him; he needs to be accepted still as part of society; he needs to be consulted in family discussions; he needs to be allowed to express himself; he expects to see his doctor daily if possible and he expects to be treated as a human being.

Care for the dying must be positive in its approach even though the outcome is realised and accepted by those who undertake this work. This is why the truths of the Passion and Resurrection are so significant; death may have concluded the earthly ministry of Our Lord, but it also opened up that glorious eternal life available for all. Acceptance of this great reality will ensure that the morbid outlook found in some nurses who say they enjoy working with the dying, does not develop. Death indeed is the moment of truth, but it should also be the moment of glorious hope; death is the one act of which we can never have prior experience and therefore the preparation can only ever be support, reassurance, compassion and understanding.

Both authors believe that care of the dying should not be regarded as a specialty. They are of the opinion that nurses and physiotherapists should have received firm grounding in basic techniques so that they can approach such patients with confidence and offer practical help. The true understanding of the spiritual and psychological needs will only be acquired through experience both with patients and their relatives and by observation and discussion with others who have worked longer in this field. The understanding of needs cannot be neatly listed in textbooks; each patient is essentially an individual and his needs have to be assessed accordingly. The student nurse will look for guidance from her seniors and the way in which she is helped and supported on the first occasion she is present at a death could well influence her approach to death for the rest of her career.

In this age of diminishing influence of religion the role of the priest is often forgotten. No priest can perform his duty to a dying patient unless he is alerted to the situation. The nurse should be aware not only of the wishes of the patient and relatives in this matter, but she should also be aware of how the particular priest wishes to be used. So often one hears of the priest being advised so late that he can only say the commendatory prayers, whereas if he had known sooner he could have helped not only the patient and family but possibly the nurses also. The care of the dying, of necessity, must be teamwork between practical caring professionals to enable the dying to live their remaining days in the certain knowledge that they will be enabled to die in peace with dignity.

Euthanasia is spoken about by well-intentioned, but often ill-informed, people. Neither author has had experience of any patient requesting such action. It is not death that people fear; it is the process of dying and the very real fear of being subjected to unpleasant treatments with no real purpose save that of satisfying medical science. If this latter fear can be confidently resolved and the patient and his family convinced and reassured that he will neither be allowed to suffer pain, nor be regarded as useless and a nuisance, then the question of euthanasia should not even be contemplated.

True care of the dying patient does not involve sophisticated medical treatments or routine examinations and blood tests; it demands nursing care of the very highest standards.

THE ROLE OF THE NURSE

It has already been stated that care of the dying demands the highest standards of nursing. The nurse's role is essentially one of caring, support, observation and anticipation.

Caring
This involves the sympathetic understanding of the patient's needs and of gentle yet firm handling in the carrying out of essential nursing techniques. It includes the all important fact of seeing that the patient and his bed are always clean and fresh;

this may mean an almost incessant changing of clothes, linen and dressings if the patient is incontinent, or has offensive and discharging wounds. Nurses need to carry out these services with patience and be able to reassure the patient that they do it willingly.

For any person, the inability to look after himself can cause much distress and feelings of shame, and it is essentially the nurse's duty to show by her caring and by the way she carries out these intimate acts, that she does it with compassion and understanding. The actual touch through handling can tell much to a patient; instinctively he knows whom he can trust, and the way in which a nurse turns or rolls a patient on to his side, or lifts him in the bed, can sometimes make or mar the nurse/patient relationship. Firm handling does not mean rough rolling; gentle handling does not mean ineffective lifting. It means the firm confident approach which instinctively conveys reassurance; it is possible to feel a patient relax if well handled.

The handling of patients also entails correct positioning of pillows; this may take a long time to achieve comfort but it is important for a patient's well-being and time spent on this is well worthwhile. Light bedclothes and bed cradles may be needed; there is nothing worse than leaving a well made bed and a beautifully washed patient, and yet making him a prisoner in his bed because his feet are pinned down by tight and heavy bedclothes and he is cold because his shoulders have no coverings over them. Dying patients do not require the strict hospital régime; commonsense and intuition and homely actions are more important.

Support

The nurse is in daily contact with her patient and her ready presence should be the support that all dying patients look to. Her support will be shown by the way she keeps the patient informed of outside activities and by the way she encourages him to make small decisions for himself. She should know the relatives and find out from them the little things that the patient likes and appreciates. Most patients have good and bad days; the good nurse supports him through the bad ones by helping him to accept that each day is a separate entity and that the bad day should be forgotten and the next one anticipated. Support for a dying patient may mean simply sitting by the bedside holding his hand. Support for the relatives may mean only listening to them; how often one hears expressed the simple words 'Thank you for listening—I feel better for having said it all.'

Observation and Anticipation

All nurses are trained to observe but this is a faculty which must be developed with experience. It cannot be taught and for the dying patient it is essential. It means looking for signs of unadmitted pain; of unmentioned worries; noting changes in the physical signs. Many patients are afraid to admit having pain because they do not want to be heavily sedated. The good nurse, having observed this, should be able to reassure the patient, report the situation to the doctor and then, by her observation, assist in resolving problems by helping to assess the level of analgesic or sedative required. No patient need ever suffer pain, but some feel they should stoically bear it; the nurse must observe and act. The worried patient is usually noticed when he thinks he is alone and unobserved; the deep sigh, the puckered brow, the clenched fist and occasionally the tears. The observant nurse will either report this to her senior, or if she feels able, will sit down by the side of the patient and try gently to find out the cause. Again the mere fact of someone, as it were, getting inside the patient and recognising the worry, may be enough for the patient to open his heart and express himself. The old saying of 'a trouble shared is a trouble halved' is very appropriate to this situation.

The nurse should endeavour to anticipate the needs of the patient; where pain is concerned she gives the prescribed drugs before the patient asks for them. She anticipates an alteration in position before the moment of discomfort arrives. All this sounds mundane, but it really is the essence of care; how often one hears a patient say 'I didn't like to ask nurse, she's so busy.' If you can anticipate, this additional worry never arises.

The role of the nurse in short is to give confidence to the patient, to be ever willing in her tasks, to be always professional and yet compassionate and finally, to accept the care of the dying as the highest test of her calling.

THE ROLE OF THE PHYSIOTHERAPIST

A number of Homes and Hospices for the dying are well aware of the great value of the physiotherapist, but alas, many physiotherapists are not willing to accept that the care of the dying is a necessary part of their work. Many so-called dying patients are transferred from active units to Homes where they can be nursed until death intervenes. All who work in these Homes know only too well, that some of these patients improve quite dramatically and can even return home for a short time. They will obviously benefit considerably from the skilled ministrations of a physiotherapist who has fashioned her own philosophy towards these patients. For the paralysed and bedridden patient, passive and active assisted movements of limbs will help the circulation and ease uncomfortable joints; massage has the dual advantage of physical help as well as providing an opportunity for the patient to talk.

It cannot be over-emphasised that one of the great requirements in care of the dying patient is giving time and being available for listening and supporting. The role of the physiotherapist is essentially in this area. The question is often asked by physiotherapists, 'What should I do if I am asked to treat a dying patient who develops pneumonia?' The answer is really simple: if by treating him with *simple* physiotherapeutic measures he is helped to be more comfortable, then proceed. If in any doubt, ask yourself whether you would wish your own parents to be treated in a similar situation. If the answer is an unqualified affirmative, then proceed. In no circumstances should this treatment cause additional distress and if the patient is unconscious, tracheal suction and physiotherapy are not justified. There must be no thought of heroic efforts to save life; the only thought must be directed to the patient's comfort and to enable him to die more peacefully.

Physiotherapy can also be used in helping nurses to handle patients with greater ease and comfort. Often the patient with advanced malignant disease may have bone metastases and nurses are afraid of handling limbs for fear they may fracture. Nothing transmits itself more readily than fear and if a nurse is afraid of handling such limbs, the patient will soon become aware of this. Firm gentle handling is necessary and often the presence of a physiotherapist, used to moving injured limbs, can give the required confidence to both nurse and patient alike. This is an area of patient care where physiotherapy and nursing can really be a profitable joint effort.

CONCLUSION

A stage is reached in a progressive illness when acceptance of the nearness of death becomes a reality and the care of the dying enters a different phase of concern. Often it causes a greater response from the patient and certainly care can become a more meaningful act. This gradual acceptance is well described by van Zeller:

'. . . it is worth noting that when people come to die they do not in fact feel the dread which has been a dark shadow to them when in the full enjoyment of life. As the faculties begin to fail there seems to be less in the temporal order to excite the sense of longing. A new norm is substituted for the old and it seems natural rather than abnormal to die. When one is in health this cannot well be imagined but when dying (such seems to be the experience) the perspectives are so altered as to make the possession of health seem remote and less real than the existing condition. Whether by a natural or supernatural dispensation the partings are accordingly eased. People who have any sense of the spiritual at all are confident that eventually they will be reunited with those from whom they are now separating, and against the interruption of human love every other letting go is as nothing. A life's work left unfinished? A place or an environment to be sacrificed? These things do not seem important any more'.

Everyone concerned with care of the progressively ill patient, through the period of dying to the point of death itself, should be able to see in it the pattern of life. Such confidence and reassurance should show itself to patient and relative in every deed and action and so enable them to be given strength to face whatever may come.

This chapter has been deliberately written from the Christian point of view; indeed it would have been impossible to do otherwise for both authors are practising Anglicans, but they equally respect the views of agnostics, humanists and others. They know that this work is a daily test of their own faith and moreover they know that many patients who are nearing the end of life are looking for something with meaning upon which they may hold. Many an unbeliever has found peace and tranquility through the knowledge that those who care for him are able to offer an indefinable extra to the routine physical care.

It is because we are Christians that we know that physical death is only the end of an earthly existence; and equally it is because of this great truth that we know that care of the dying is in reality learning to live. Dr R. C. Mortimer, formerly Bishop of Exeter, described so vividly the act of death and the theology of Body and Soul that we quote his words:

'. . . The Soul which entered the body at the moment of conception, which gives "form" to the body, and in which Christians believe, is a subservient spiritual entity which can survive the dissolution of its union with the body. It is this dissolution which we call Death; of the Soul, we know by faith, that it is in the hands of its merciful Creator who prepares for it a "spiritual" body wherein and wherewith it can worship and serve the Creator in that Glorious "risen" life, which it was from the beginning destined and created to enjoy'.

It is this glorious, triumphant hope that should give strength not only to those who work in the peaceful havens where men and women are lovingly cared for, encouraged and prepared for that final step into the Great Unknown, but also to the patients who are entrusted to their care. Few will be able to say with Pope John, 'I am ready, my bags are packed'; all could pray with St Francis of Assisi:

> And thou most kind and gentle death,
> Waiting to hush our latest breath,
> Thou leadest home the child of God,
> And Christ our Lord, the way has trod.[1]

ACKNOWLEDGEMENT

The authors are deeply grateful to Dr R. C. Mortimer, D.D., and *The Sunday Times*, and to Dom Hubert van Zeller and Messrs.

[1]Trs. W. H. Draper, 'All creatures of Our God and King', Hymn based on St Francis of Assisi's Canticle of the Sun, Hymns A & M Revised, 172.

Sheed and Ward for permission to quote from their works. They also acknowledge that without the support of patients over many years these impressions would not have been possible.

REFERENCES

Graeme, P. D. (1975) *Support for the dying patient and his family.* In The Marie Curie Memorial Foundation Symposium on Cancer, the Patient and the Family (Ed. Raven, R. W.). Altrincham: John Sherratt & Son.
Guardini, R. (1954) *The Last Things.* London: Burns & Oates.
Mortimer, R. C. (1962) Union with the Soul. *The Sunday Times*, March 18.
Van Zeller, H. (1973) *Leave Your Life Alone.* London: Sheed & Ward.

13

Relief of Pain and Stress

D. S. ROBBIE

PAIN AND STRESS are known to us all. Some fortunate people manage to pass through their lives with little of either, but in our Westernised society the impinging stresses are increasingly taking their toll.

Pain is a very common symptom. Doctors are trained to find out the cause of the pain rather than deal with the symptom. However, in many cases all that can be done is to treat the pain symptomatically. If the pain is transient, sub-optimal treatment is not a heavy burden for the patient. Unfortunately the symptom is often chronic and intractable and the disease process unable to be subdued or cured. In these unfortunate circumstances it is important that the doctor should be optimal in his treatment of the symptom. Optimal treatment inevitably varies with the environment in which the doctor and patient find themselves, for instance their access to drugs and hospitals. There is little doubt that the best treatment available is often not given.

The symptomatic treatment of pain by various methods is dealt with in this chapter. Obviously pain may disappear with the specific treatment of a disease process, but this is not discussed here.

Stress is part of life and feeds on the discomfort of pain, increasing each in an upward spiral. Thus the doctor and his helpers must aim to prevent and reduce the upward spiral of stress, particularly when this is associated with pain. The less well either symptom is managed, the less well the patient will be both symptomatically and generally.

PAIN
USE OF THE ANALGESICS

The hard fact of medical care is that most patients will only be offered drugs for their pain, which are the most important single item of treatment. However, the intelligent use of available drugs leaves much to be desired. Pain is very common and most people either ignore it or take a remedy bought from a retailer. Many pains will settle with this régime.

There are many drugs to relieve physical pain (analgesics) and the commonest is aspirin. This is very effective, especially if used by adults in doses of up to 1 g every four hours. Some patients may suffer a gastrointestinal upset with aspirin, but they often fear this without justification. On inquiry one may find that the favourite home analgesic is aspirin alone or in combination under a trade name. There is concern at the risk of any major gastrointestinal bleeding and also of steady small amounts of blood loss if the aspirin is being taken regularly over a long period of time in chronic conditions. To try to minimise such side effects aspirin is marketed in many different forms intended to be less irritant to the gastrointestinal tract, but shielded forms of aspirin may be less efficacious if they are less well absorbed from the intestine than the unshielded drug. There is concern that aspirin, like other mild analgesics, may cause kidney damage, but this is an open question at present, compared with the general condemnation of the chronic use of phenacetin because of its nephrotoxic properties. Nevertheless, large quantities of aspirin are taken every day and no absolute ban on it has yet been suggested because of the incidence of side effects.

It may be prudent to try other analgesics in the first instance and continue with them instead of aspirin if they are satisfactory. Paracetamol is a suitable drug to try first as a general analgesic. Adults usually take 1 g every four hours as required. Paracetamol is considered to be safer than aspirin especially with regard to gastrointestinal bleeding and there is no real concern about nephrotoxic properties at present. The clinical position is that a smaller percentage of patients will obtain satisfactory analgesia from paracetamol than from aspirin. If it does not give relief, a less irritant (shielded) form of aspirin can be tried.

Codeine is rarely used by itself as an analgesic, but is often added to aspirin and/or paracetamol in the hope of an enhanced analgesic effect from the combination. In the doses used the codeine may not have a very worthwhile analgesic action and it causes constipation, especially when taken regularly.

Dextropopoxyphene is used widely as an analgesic, alone, or in combination with other analgesics, such as paracetamol. There is no good evidence that dextropopoxyphene is a satisfactory analgesic alone and the good effects of a combination with paracetamol are probably mainly those of paracetamol. Clinically, some branded combinations seem to be liked and found effective by patients, perhaps because they like the shape of the tablet and/or the tablets slide down easily.

These commonly used analgesics may not be satisfactory either because of insufficient analgesia or unwanted side effects. The next up the strength scale are two commonly prescribed analgesics, dihydrocodeine and pentazocine.

Dihydrocodeine is taken orally in doses of 30 to 60 mg. It is a drug with some addictive potential but this is regarded as less than that of the opiates. It certainly is more powerful than the milder analgesics, but it can cause unpleasant side effects. The most noticeable of these are feelings of light-headedness, drowsiness and marked constipation. Here, as with all drugs, one has to consider the situation in which the patient is taking the drug. If the patient is immobilised in a hospital bed the mental side effects may be tolerable, but when mobile he may be incapacitated by these side effects and a danger to all. Again, the manufacturers try to reach a compromise by combining smaller doses of dihydrocodeine with paracetamol.

Pentazocine is a more recent introduction available as tablets, capsules and suppositories and for injection. It is claimed to be a powerful analgesic with minimal abuse potential. The worst side effects on the central nervous system are light-headedness with unpleasant or pleasant feelings and sometimes hallucinations. It is possible to become 'attached' to the pleasant mental effects. With ambulant patients a satisfactory analgesic dose may not avoid these psychotomimetic effects. Again, these effects are less noticeable in the recumbent patient.

Pentazocine is a mild antagonist of morphine-like drugs and the position is not clear in clinical practice, whether it is wise either to combine it or alternate it with morphine-like drugs, lest analgesia is lessened rather than enhanced as intended. Certainly, in patients who have been having significant doses of opiates for some time, injections of pentazocine can cause morphine withdrawal symptoms.

The next step in analgesic escalation is drugs that are regarded as 'hard' and have a significant abuse and addiction potential. These include the most powerful analgesics. Possibly, pethidine is the most freely prescribed drug in this group. It was introduced as a non-addictive drug and received a tremendous boost from this claim which we now know is incorrect. However, attitudes and habits are slow to alter and pethidine is much more freely prescribed than morphine, and allowed to be used by midwives virtually on their own initiative. Pethidine is not a good oral analgesic; when given by mouth and particularly by injection it can cause unpleasant mental sensations of non-well-being (dysphoria).

There are many other morphine substitute drugs on the market. Phenazocine is used both as tablets and injection and is worth a trial.

For any patient, one may have to use many different analgesics to find the most suitable one. An open mind is necessary in surveillance of the drug administration and change to another analgesic required if the current one appears ineffective even in larger doses. The patient may develop a drug tolerance, or the pain may be increasing in severity. This type of progression must be very much in the mind of the prescriber dealing with patients dying in pain from incurable cancer.

Dipipanone is available in combination with an anti-emetic to help counteract the fairly common gastrointestinal side effects of powerful analgesics and may be useful.

Another strong analgesic that is used commonly is dextromoramide. A number of clinicians have found this drug to be addictive and not particularly effective in chronic cancer pain, and it is not recommended for use in chronic pain.

Methadone in doses of 5–10 mg is a very effective oral analgesic, and is usually worth trying for severe pain, especially in the terminal phase of cancer. Occasionally nausea, vomiting or drowsiness occur, and as with most of these drugs, costiveness may be a problem. The efficacy of methadone is highlighted by its value as a substitute for heroin in régimes aiming to withdraw heroin in addicts.

The strongest analgesics available for general use are morphine and heroin (diamorphine). Heroin is prescribed in very few countries now because of the great concern about problems of abuse and drug-dependence as socio-economic evils. Heroin was nearly banned in the United Kingdom about twenty years ago but this was stopped because a group of eminent clinicians felt strongly that it had a number of advantages over morphine which were irreplaceable. There is still a strong clinical impression that heroin has advantages over morphine both orally and by injection because of the lesser side effects of nausea, vomiting, constipation and dysphoria. Nevertheless, because of the abuse problem, doctors in this country are much less ready to prescribe morphine and especially heroin than in the past. Heroin has one outstanding physical advantage in being much more soluble than morphine; it is available in ampoules as a freeze-dried powder which mixes readily with small amounts of water. In the relatively common severe pain caused by incurable cancer, especially when there is vomiting, frequent injections of large doses of heroin can be given regularly in small amounts of solution. This is of great advantage in a wasted patient who may need many injections. Heroin is usually regarded as having twice the strength of morphine by injection.

More commonly for the terminal cancer pain morphine and/or heroin are given orally and it is essential to give a sufficient dose often enough to relieve the pain. Tablets of the drugs can be used, or simple solutions may be preferred. More often euphoriant mixtures are prepared which also contain in each dose cocaine 10 mg and gin 4 ml. An orange flavouring is often less sickly than syrup or honey. These mixtures should be tailored to the patient, for instance it may be found either suitable or unsatisfactory to give gin to a life-long teetotaller; only trial and error will tell.

There is a tendency to use eponymous names for these euphoriant mixtures, especially in hospital, and often the medical and nursing staff are unaware of the exact doses and ingredients of the mixture. This limits their accurate assessment of the effects, especially for further prescribing of drugs for the patient.

Morphine is often added to aspirin and paracetamol mixtures for cancer pain in the form of 'Nepenthe'. It is not often realised that each ml of 'Nepenthe' contains 8 mg of morphine and the attitude of prescribing may be more relaxed than intended. Such mixtures are very potent analgesics, but tend to be nauseous and constipating. Not surprisingly they seem to be quite addictive in clinical practice.

The above represents a selection of analgesic drugs which may deal with the problem of physical pain as it presents. However, there are many pains that respond only partly or not at all to analgesics. This is not to suggest that they are not real to the patient or do occur, but they do not respond to analgesics alone. They are fairly described as unpleasant sensations (dysaesthesias) and may be partly relieved more by the simpler rather than the stronger analgesics. Many of these patients sleep well at night, and if distracted by something pleasurable, such as a favourite television programme, will temporarily forget their pain. This type of dysaesthesia can be felt in areas that have been mutilated by surgery, in the scar tissue either on the skin surface or deeper. The classic syndrome of phantom pain after an amputated limb is well known. A common dysaesthesia is post-herpetic neuralgia which is most common in elderly patients and has an above average incidence in certain types of cancer, e.g. lymphoma and leukaemia.

With constant chronic pain it is vital to emphasise to the patient that the pain relieving drugs must be taken regularly, which may mean every four hours. We know that it is easier to keep pain at bay by adequate doses given regularly. It may be necessary to use larger than maintenance doses at first to subdue the severe pain.

Again, patients may have relatively little pain at bedrest but this is exacerbated by movement. They must have adequate sedation before movement so that the drugs have time to be absorbed and act. Effective potent short-acting analgesics are not readily available for general use and most drugs seem to act for about four hours in the correct dose.

It must be recognised that some patients are very reluctant to take drugs, and it is impossible to alter this attitude. This can be accentuated by the tendency of all drugs, especially analgesics, to costiveness, and this is a very human and sometimes obsessional concern of many patients. Ill, wasted patients with poor appetites do not eat the food necessary for a good bowel movement, but the defaecating habit is very entrenched. Sympathetic attention to the bowels is vital to get the patient feeling well and ready to take effective analgesics. Aperients such as liquid paraffin preparations, taken regularly through the day may be more logical than larger amounts at night.

In patients who will not take analgesics it may be that some other technical method should be considered.

Patients should sleep at night both for their own comfort and the relief of attending relatives. Of course the desire to sleep at night is often less if the patient sleeps for periods during the day. However, in chronic severe pain it is important to give effective analgesics throughout the night as well.

It is found there is minimal drowsiness from opiates in the treatment of severe pain as opposed to the patient without pain who has side effects from opiates given, for example, as a pre-medication to surgery. However, if drowsiness is a problem the use of cerebral stimulant drugs to cover the times of desired awakeness can be valuable. Amphetamines are the standard drugs of this type, but there are many substitutes, and long acting preparations of both groups are available to act throughout the day.

SOME SPECIFIC DRUG TREATMENTS

Arthritic Diseases

Many dying patients have arthritis of different varieties and the associated pains may respond to the many specific anti-arthritic drugs that are available. Unfortunately, as with all drugs, the side effects may be worse than the disease or the benefits of the drug, and the drug régime needs careful supervision for maximum benefit.

In practice it is found that patients dying from widespread cancer, especially when the bones are involved, respond significantly to the anti-inflammatory drugs and their use should be actively considered and tried in suitable circumstances.

Trigeminal Neuralgia

This unfortunate ailment is not uncommon in the dying patient and may respond well to specific drugs based on carbamazepine. However, it has not been found that other forms of neuralgia or pain have an encouraging response to carbamazepine.

TECHNICAL PROCEDURES FOR THE SYMPTOMATIC RELIEF OF PAIN

Doctors have striven by various means to interrupt the nerve fibres that carry pain. This has been done in a number of ways over the years and new methods are continuously being investigated and assessed.

Nerve Blocking with Chemical Solutions

Perhaps the oldest, simplest and most commonly used attempts to relieve pain involve the use of local anaesthetic solutions on one or several occasions in the hope of breaking the so-called vicious circle or spiral of the pain process. The great attraction of this method is that the effects of the local anaesthetic are reversible and any ill effects should be minimal. As one might expect, the good effects are limited.

Many attempts are made to strengthen the chemicals to produce a more lasting local anaesthetic effect. A variety of nerve damaging (neurolytic) drugs have been used, but the commonest have been solutions of alcohol (50–100 per cent), and solutions of phenol (4–10 per cent) in a heavy solution such as glycerine. Stronger solutions of phenol (25 per cent) are used to damage motor function in situations where there is a spastic paraplegia. The spastic state of the muscles is replaced by flaccidity and nursing care in bed is much easier and more efficient. The patient is more comfortable in bed, and may now be able to sit in a chair for long periods which is advantageous for all. Even a weaker solution damages all the nerve fibres it contacts to such an extent that balanced judgement must be made about the risks of good and bad effects and the acceptability to the patient of the latter. This must take into consideration that the dying patient has usually little superficial frank insight into his prognosis which increases any recrimination about the deficits produced.

In recent years there have been introduced, or re-introduced, techniques where the hope is for good benefit with little or no deficit. However, there is no general agreement as to their place at present. These include the use of intrathecal hypertonic saline and the pumping to and fro of the cerebrospinal fluid, sometimes after cooling it.

The value of nerve blocking might best be illustrated by the following three examples:

Case 1

An elderly lady had disseminated cancer and was bedridden. She had a swollen leg and a very painful knee due to metastases.

While still in bed her pain was fairly readily controlled, but she was a large woman and required nursing care several times a day to her pressure areas. This was excruciatingly painful for her, so much so that she required very large doses of intramuscular diamorphine to allow the nursing care to be carried out. Even then it was a trial for all and a recurring painful experience for the patient. She had an attentive circle of family and friends with good *rapport*, but the high dose of analgesic required for the excruciating pain of moving the knee kept her very drowsy after she returned to the relatively pain-free recumbent bed position, therefore the mental and physical *rapport* was frustrated. She already had an indwelling catheter, so there was no need for concern about urinary control. Also, she required manual disimpaction of faeces twice a week, which was no additional problem. She was unable to walk, so there was no anxiety about deficit in ambulation following the nerve block. Therefore, she had a spinal aneasthetic under a general anaesthetic (because of the pain) as a trial of treatment and was completely relieved of her painful knee for some hours. Subsequently a strong injection of phenol was given into her cerebrospinal fluid, again under general anaesthesia and there was very satisfactory relief of pain in her knee for the subsequent few months of her life. She still required smaller doses of diamorphine for general pain control, but her mental state was absolutely satisfactory for her social contacts.

Case 2

An elderly lady was admitted to hospital with a very painful arm due to cancer spreading into the brachial plexus in her neck. She found she became dizzy with strong analgesics and disliked taking them anyway. It was possible to inject the brachial plexus with a solution of phenol in alcohol which relieved her severe pain for a month and allowed her to go home and manage with some assistance. After a month there was some recurrence of pain and the injection was repeated which allowed her again to return home and die there some weeks later in a relatively pain-free state and mentally clear to the end.

Case 3

A young woman had incurable cancer in her upper abdomen and severe upper abdominal pain which required her hospitalisation and the injection of opiates to control the pain. She had a local anaesthetic block of her coeliac plexus (sympathetic nerves). This greatly relieved her pain and so a block with alcohol was carried out. This was successful and remained effective until her death three months later. She was able to be maintained pain-free at home with oral analgesics. The only side effect was some light-headedness on sitting up, which lasted for a few days immediately after the block.

Neurosurgery

Naturally the surgeon is concerned with cutting the nerve tracts carrying pain to solve some of these problems. Again, the balance of benefit and deficit is real and has to be judged for each individual patient.

The classical established operation for the treatment of intractable pain is mid-thoracic section of the antero-lateral spino-thalamic tract on the opposite side to the pain. This gives unilateral relief below the umbilicus, but involves the major surgical operation of laminectomy. Many dying patients are not fit enough for this procedure, or their prognosis does not warrant the attempt. Sections above the thoracic region by open surgery carry a high morbidity and mortality.

To overcome the major risk of laminectomy it is possible to damage the antero-lateral spino-thalamic tract high in the neck by a needle inserted under radiological control without general anaesthesia. This procedure can be repeated if necessary, but is so far not readily available throughout the United Kingdom.

Newer techniques are being assessed where electrical stimulus to the dorsal (sensory) columns of the spinal cord relieves pain. It is too early to know how practically and realistically helpful these will be.

Other Surgery

It would be incomplete not to note that in cancer of the breast relief of pain and regression of disease can follow endocrine ablation by oophorectomy, adrenalectomy and hypophysectomy. Some benefit may occur solely with the use of steroid drugs.

Palliative surgery to relieve distress in the dying may be very valuable, for example, to by-pass obstructions in the gastro-intestinal tract.

Radiotherapy

Radiotherapy is often of benefit in relieving the pain of incurable cancer by retarding or destroying the metastatic tumour cells. This is classically the case in osseous metastases from breast cancer, but it is valuable to consider radiotherapy right through the whole range of tissue accessible to radiation therapy where the side effects are acceptable. Benefit can accrue in localised areas with relatively radio-resistant tumours, such as rectal cancer in the sacral plexus area.

Cytotoxic (Anti-mitotic) Drugs

One of the palliative indications for the use of cytotoxic drugs is in localised pain. Sometimes the drug can be delivered exactly by intra-arterial cannulation, but where this is not possible, oral or intravenous cytotoxic mixtures may be very beneficial with tolerable side effects from treatment.

STRESS

We are all aware there is mental reaction, often of a stressful nature, to all our actions and efforts. The dying situation is self-evidently stressful, affecting all involved. It is not uncommon for the mental stress to be partially or totally ignored to the distress of the patient, relatives and associates. It is particularly in these circumstances that it may seem easier to the patient to complain of an orthodox symptom such as pain which gains them attention and sympathy. Very often the complaint is accepted without any sensible enquiry and is treated by medication. The patient obtains misdirected superficial attention that rarely satisfies the stress.

THE TABOO

Much has been said and written about the knowledge of patients concerning their condition. I can only speak from my own professional and general experience. It seems that it is very rare for the patient to be accurately or sympathetically appraised of his condition or prognosis, and this applies very often to close relatives as well. This excludes the group of patients and relatives who reject the facts offered.

The axis of the patient and the doctor is moulded by the

personality of each and the *rapport* established between them. The problems of maintaining the same doctor/patient relationship in general practice and hospital seem legion, and sometimes are not even desirable with the personalities involved.

With the cancer patient the taboo in the United Kingdom seems pre-eminent. These patients will very often have seen many doctors of all levels of seniority in several different specialities and can end up as lost creatures. The most satisfying link with their situation may be through a particular nurse, a member of the ancillary staff, or social worker, and little concern is shown or appreciated for the distress and frustration that the non-doctor personnel can suffer in this situation.

MANAGEMENT

Human Support
This is the most critical and essential way to diminish stress. The vital factor is time. It is true that some time must be spent with the doctors, but usually not a great deal. The senior doctor when involved must also spend a minimum time to carry on the support bandwagon.

Thus, time and talk are essential. It will depend on the patient whether talking or listening is more vital at any one time. Again, one has to be realistic in the economical use of trained talents, and here less skilled volunteer workers can develop a great value.

It is, of course, a simple form of psychotherapy and does need some direction, liaison and discussion by the staff involved to be maximally beneficial. This will apply whatever environment the patient is in, home, acute or chronic hospital. In some terminal institutions with good staffing, a bridge has been established between the home and the hospital by hospital staff visiting the domestic scene as necessary. The patient can be admitted or re-admitted to the hospital as necessary on an acute or chronic basis, but will be maintained at home as much as possible, which is obviously a socio-economic benefit.

In institutions caring for the dying there is no doubt that the nursing orientation, efficiency and vocation is much more readily achieved to a higher standard than general hospitalisation. Similarly the attending medical staff can give their time whole-heartedly to the problems of the dying. This does not in any way recommend isolation from the centres of therapy which may be desirable during the terminal illness. It is much easier to organise suitable diversional and occupational activities in a terminal home.

The problem of the death rate in terminal homes has not proved to be a formidable obstacle to satisfactory and acceptable care and mental tranquillity. The expertise in dealing with the problems is pre-eminently successful.

Drug Support

It is fashionable to forget old, cheap drugs, but they are often helpful and certainly under-used in modern pharmaceutical surroundings. The benefits of small regular doses of phenobarbitone are almost forgotten today. The excellent stimulant uses of the amphetamines have fallen under the long twin shadows of abuse and dependence, and strong pressure groups would wish their total withdrawal, presumably making way for more expensive and possibly less desirable substitutes. There is evidence that the analgesic effect of opiates is enhanced by amphetamines.

In the really late and occasional unsupportable stages of dying, intramuscular phenobarbitone, probably used with effective opiate doses, can be a tranquil blessing compared with many drugs in use.

There is a plethora of competing psychotropic drugs which are the current panacea for many ills. Usually their side effects are minimised in selling them and no sooner have we become familiar with the uses and limitations of one set of drugs than another new more expensive patented product is presented as upstaging all present drugs. Often it takes years before the lie becomes evident, but usually at the least a substantial financial gain has been made by the drug firm concerned. We are rarely considering use of the psychotropic drugs available in the doses used in psychiatric practice, but in doses up to those used in the most extreme anxieties dealt with in general practice.

Diazepam has almost become the best known drug of recent years. It is a tranquilliser with sedative effects and some value in decreasing muscular spasm. In fact, diazepam can be a very successful hypnotic. Small doses, 2 mg, are often ignored for bigger doses with undesirable sedative effects.

Chlordiazepoxide has been used for a long time as a tranquilliser and is still used widely in mild anxiety. The sedative side effects are less noticeable than with diazepam.

Amitriptyline, a well-established tricyclic drug, has been found useful, especially for difficult dysaesthesias. It can be used in a single dose at night when there is a hypnotic action and the anti-anxiety and anti-depression action continues throughout the day. Usual doses are 100 mg but more may be required. Sometimes patients seem to have sleepy side effects with lesser doses. Tricyclic drugs can cause urinary retention and constipation and may have to be withdrawn in sensitive patients. In psychiatry bigger doses of the tricyclic drugs may be recommended and it is said that the good effects take some weeks to develop. However, in the control of pain smaller doses seem to be effective and sometimes work quite rapidly. This does not appear to be a placebo effect.

Chlorpromazine is an established drug used widely in severe cancer pain together with opiates. However, the side effects of chlorpromazine, particularly drowsiness, are often distressing to the patient and it is probably required less often than it is used. It is often prescribed before effective analgesics have been fully tried in high enough dosage or given frequently enough.

Terminal cancer patients with pain often benefit from steroids. These give rise to feelings of well-being, increase the appetite and a little water retention will lessen the weight loss noticed by the patient. Doses may start with prednisone 5–10 mg twice a day, but larger doses may be beneficial and have little ill effect.

Material Support

It is evident there may be severe financial stresses associated with the dying patient. This is particularly so with the young patient dying from cancer, who is the bread-winner or mother of young children. We must be prepared and proselytise for sufficient financial support to enable as normal a social pattern to continue as is possible. The knowledge of this support will greatly reassure the dying patient.

Religious Support

In modern society, particularly in the urban and metropolitan scenes, there has been a complete disruption of settled patterns and modes of life that have succoured people over the centuries. The comparative absence of the romantic family doctor presence and the lessening of religious community have left many people in a vacuum which the modern state social services are incompetent to fill.

There is no doubt it is essential for suitable religious support to be available for the dying patient, although preferably not to be pressed by priest and family on an unwilling patient.

There is also a lack of doctor/priest *rapport* which should be strengthened for the benefit of the patient and family and would be helpful in their own work.

COMMENT

There is no doubt that in the United Kingdom during the last decade there has been an increasing amount of work and thought about the care of the dying. In particular there is great concern to prevent unnecessary pain, especially in incurable cancer. We are far from an optimal position in the use of even the analgesic drugs, but education by example has and will increase this basic comfort to patients.

Increasingly, the stressful side of all medical, social and community problems is being recognised although the remedies are often beyond the willingness of the masses (and their governments) to sustain financially, morally or personally. However, the guide lines are being laid down and clarified for further improvement in these fields.

Index